The Perfect Life Diet

For Imperfect People With Weight Problems

Introducing: The Dieters Scale ©
&
The Human Dynamics Matrix for Weight Problems ©

An Original Work Created and Developed By:

David John Sheridan

aka Guru David

When you know better; you can do better!

Updated May 2021

ISBN-978-0-9932355-3-5

DEDICATION

I dedicate this book to all those great people whose lives are being blighted and destroyed by a persistent weight problem.

A Persistent weight problem can cast a shadow over someone's life and rob their life of happiness.

I want to help people move out of the shadow of a persistent weight problem and into the sunshine of the life that they want to live.

To do this I have been working for many years to develop better, higher quality, more reliable and innovative solutions. Focused on helping people achieve successful results with persistent weight problems and other types of problems.

When we are talking about Weight Control, Dieting, Exercise and Lifestyle Management; we are talking about a big and complex subject. This is an area which contains a lot of difficult issues; which can also be complicated

There is also a lot of confusion, mythology and false and misleading information in this area.

If we are going to successfully deal with persistent weight problems we have to accept the reality that a weight problem impacts our lives and that our lives impact a weight problem.

We can achieve the successful changes we want

by working together. So follow me; we need to go in this direction!

A Persistent Weight Problem is a set of conditions looking for a better way of being managed, so as to produce a more successful result.

Guru David
David John Sheridan

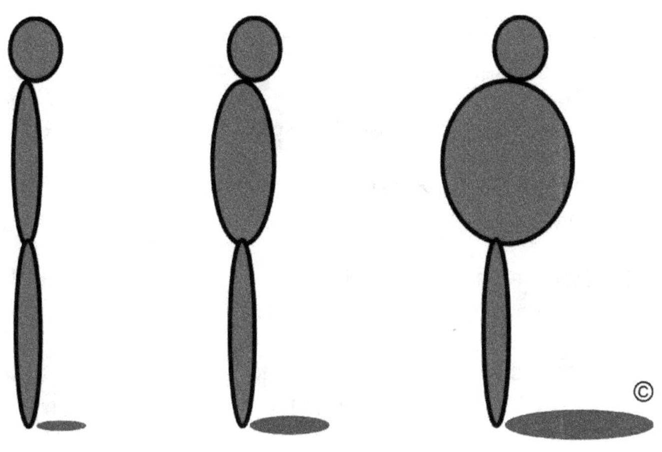

Too Thin! **Too Fat!**

Extremely Negative ← Normal Range → Extremely Positive

The Spectrum of Weight Problems

CONTENTS

	Acknowledgements	ix
1	Introduction.	1
2	Imperfect People.	18
3	Where Are You On The Dieters Scale?	28
4	The Best And Most Successful Diet In The World.	46
5	Eat When You Want; Just Accept The Consequences.	55
6	Food Addiction – Fact Or Myth?	66
7	Permanently Changing Your Life Profile for Food, etc.	95
8	Stop Measuring The Symptom: Your Weight. And Start Measuring Other Things.	103
9	Genetic Realities. Is Your Mind Writing Cheques Your Body Can't Pay!	112
10	Finding Your Seed Of Belief!	119
11	Chaos, Chaotic Behaviour and Chaotic Situations.	128
12	You Can't Walk Far When You Are Deep In A Hole.	134
13	The Reality Of Failure.	144
14	The Role Of Habits In Your Problem.	149

15	The Role Of Relationships In Your Problem.	158
16	The Role Of A Lack Of Understanding In Your Problem.	167
17	The Role Of Symptom Solutioning In Your Problem.	171
18	The Role Of Food In Your Problem.	179
19	The Role Of Processed Foods In Your Problem.	189
20	The Role Of Exercise In Your Problem.	206
21	The Role Of Influencing Factors In Your Problem.	228
22	Problems With Different Time Frames.	235
23	Body Dysmorphia And Social And General Dysmorphia.	241
24	Going Through "The Shredder".	248
25	Are You A Secret Eater, Boozer, In Denial.	252
26	An Introduction To The Human Dynamics Matrix.	257
27	Putting It All Together.	266
28	Choose Who, What And How You Want To Be; From Now On!	269
29	The Real Timeline For Becoming The Person You Want To Be.	274
30	Life Improvement Programmes.	278

Contents

31	Lifestyle, Wealth, Health & Well-Being.	283
32	Diet, Weight Loss And Exercise Classes.	293
	About Guru David.	309

Other Books by Guru David and published by Sheridan Publishing include:

For Adults

Weight Control The Hi-Way

From FAT To SLIM In 3 Steps

The Perfect Life Diet For Imperfect People With Weight Problems

Motivate & Inspire Yourself; To Do Something Positive

Self-Esteem For Imperfect People

An Introduction To The Human Dynamics Matrix

The Way of Vartis

For Children

The Magic Mustachio and the tale of The Bear That Loved Pies

Soon to follow: Oscar the sheep and the Magic Mustachio

These books are based on The Human Algorithm® Approach to understanding and working with complex and challenging problems; many of which are Psycho-somatic in structure.

ACKNOWLEDGMENTS

I have wanted to write this book for a long time.

Now that the first edition of this book is completed I would like to thank all the women that I have met through the years; who were unhappy with their weight, the way that their bodies looked and how this made them feel.

I would also like to thank them for the massive passive education that I achieved from listening to their stories.

Their tales of diets, exercises, fads, fashions and their extreme behaviours; so as to look and feel better were a real education.

I would also like to thank all those people that I met, trained with, taught and learned from in various Dojo's, training halls and gyms where we shared the world of Martial Arts.

I would like to thank those people who taught me and helped me to discover persistence, dogged determination and the ability to keep going when others would have given up.

With thanks to:

Dr Loi Lee.
Mr Bill Wright.
Mr Michael Finn
And my students and fellow travellers.

We Begin!

CHAPTER 1

INTRODUCTION

I first began professionally working with people who had weight problems in the early 1990's.

I set up a small clinic working with a number of people who had long dieting histories.

The people I worked with had all tried multiple diets and different types of weight control and exercise programmes. Some of these were main stream solutions and others were not.

At the time I was also working with various people in the area of drug and alcohol addictions. The medical team I was attached to were dealing with the very problematic and chaotic people who required a clinical detox to break the addiction cycle.

I have the sort of mind that is wired differently to most other people. I tend to see things in ways that other people don't and I tend to see things that other people tend to miss.

I am also curious, innovative, creative and quite smart.

As I was working with these different groups of people I could see patterns and structures within their behaviours.

I also saw that there were patterns and structures within their abilities to understand and manage their problems better.

I found that these patterns and structures were the same across the different conditions; drugs, alcohol, weight and other problem groups.

I realised that as well as having common factors in these conditions. That when we looked at other problems that involved people, that these common factors continued.

And over time I began to look at other types of problems where people were involved. This included businesses and social structures as these provide the frameworks within which we live and work.

My belief that there was room for new approaches for understanding and working with problems grew, as I spent more time talking to people and working with people who provided solutions to problems.

I could see that there was room to change, improve and develop new ways of understanding and working with problems that involve people.

The problem is that when you begin to connect different conditions together, you come up against different groups who specialise in those conditions.

Experts in different fields don't like "Outsiders" having and expressing views that may effect their specialisation.

Even when the Outsiders views may help them; you still encounter resistance and even hostility.

It's just the way that the system and the people behave when they are faced with new thinking.

As a result of my curiosity; I had began a process of trying to understand the architectures and structures of problems and solutions.

I wanted to understand what it was about these structures that goes on to produce the Patterns of Success and Failure and created problems.

I realised that if you could influence a Problem and a Solution in the right way, at the right time; that you could begin to produce predictable positive results.

And I realised that if I could find a way of working with all these common components that I could then work effectively with any problem that involved people; regardless of the nature of the problem!

Because of my curiosity; I began working on new ways of looking at and understanding the actual structure of problems and the solutions that they required.

What I was interested in was getting to the DNA level and understanding it from that level upwards.

I did not know that it would take me this long or that so much hard work would be involved.

This book has been written as a result of those many years of hard work and experiences.

Over the years that I have been doing this; I have developed an eye for the Patterns of Success and Failure.

Those Patterns of Success and Failure are not as obvious as we may think they are.

> Often Success is achieved by contra thinking and contra behaviour: Going against the tide rather than allowing yourself to be carried by it.

Real Success has a Philosophy. I will be sharing this Positive Life Philosophy with you.

I also want to share my insights and understanding of the structures which lead to success, with as many people as I can.

This is the type of book that you can read more than once. At each reading you may find something new and take something different that may help you understand, clarify and being working with an aspect of your life in a new way.

Take from this book what you need but try to keep an open mind to any parts of it that you find difficult.

> Almost everyone with a persistent weight problem can do something positive about it; if they go with the solution rather than the problem.

So let's begin to focus this book on improving Persistent Weight Problems.

Each of us is given a Golden Opportunity in life.

Unfortunately many of us lose our way and we get distracted away from the Golden Opportunity.

Different aspects of life get in the way and our lives can get away from us.

Changing aspects of our lives which have become broken, confused, unwanted and harmful; can be desirable but difficult to achieve.

I work in the arena of difficult, confusing, harmful and unwanted problems.

I also work in the arena of success, achieving desired outcomes, changing in positive ways and Being Truly Successful In Life.

As a Philosophical Problem Solver I look at problems to see if there are another ways of looking at and understanding them.

I also see if there are other ways of finding and applying better solutions to those problems.

Then I see how we can use that knowledge to work out the Path that we need to take, to get to the Solution that we want.

And I do this with Weight Problems.

For those with persistent weight problems the Solution seems obvious; blindingly obvious!

They want to achieve and maintain a better weight.

And we have an entire industry of diets, diet clubs, weight lose programmes, counsellors, therapist and advisers; who focus on achieving this outcome.

And yet; the problem, like the people, is growing in size and complexity.

I think that it is time to stop trying the same old solutions and let's take another look at this thing.

The problem with Persistent Weight Problems is that they are not straight-forwards.

For a start we have different types of people, different types of bodies, different ages, different sexes, different abilities and different resources.

Then we have the pressures that people bring to the Weight Problem.

They want to lose weight quickly, easily, with no exercise, with exercise, change their shape, be toned, have a younger looking body, etc.

And then we can bring in the "Other Problems".

This is the complicated mix of personal, domestic, work, social and other problems that populate the lives of people with persistent weight problems.

People with persistent weight problems are not unique when it comes to “Other Problems”.

All of us has this entourage of Other Problems which annoy and frustrate us as we move through life.

In fact we all have the same problem of:

> How do I have a better quality of life and begin living the life that I really want to live?

Through writing this book. I would like to see if I can help you to move in the right direction and do the right things; so that you can get on the Path to the real results that you want.

I would like to help you find your way back to the Golden Opportunity and help you understand and begin to deal with the persistent weight problem and the other problems that you have.

I invite you, as someone who diets, to make this the beginning of a new style of Living and Being; where you can deal with the realities of Life without turning to food to provide the help and support that you need.

Instead you will use the new tools and structures that are available for you, to help you have a better quality and more successful life in the future.

This book is going to be different from the other diet, weight reduction and exercise books that you may have read and heard about.

In this book we are going to be looking at and working with weight problems by understanding what weight problems really are.

Issues we will look at include:

- Food Addiction. Fact or Myth?
- The Best and Most Successful Diet in the World. And how you can make use of this.
- Using The Dieters Scale© to understand your problem better.

We will look at the physical, emotional, psychological and social components of a weight problem.

At the same time we will be looking at how to effectively deal with them, so that you can have a better quality of life without all the dieting pressures and disappointments.

Don't think of this process as giving you all the answers and providing you with a quick result.

Think of this as the beginning of the end of your weight problem; and the start of a new Life Opportunity for you.

You might think that you already know what a persistent weight problem really is; but in truth I doubt that you really do.

You have probably had what most people with weight problems have had:

> The experiences of having a persistent weight problem and trying many different things to deal with that weight problem.

However; this is different from understanding the problem so that you can effectively deal with it long term.

> The Experiencing of a weight problem is different from Understanding the weight problem that you are Experiencing.
>
> For example:
>
> We are all capable of eating a great meal, but just because we can eat a great meal; it doesn't mean that we now know and understand how to produce a great meal.

What I am going to do within this book is try and help you Understand your persistent weight problem and Understand how to deal with it effectively in the short and long term.

To help me do this, I am going to put weight problems into "A Spectrum of Weight Problems".

A Spectrum is simply grouping all the different

types of weight problems together and putting them side by side in a line and looking at the way that they line up and fit together.

This process helps us to see weight problems in different ways and it helps us to see commonalities, relationships and differences between the different parts of the Spectrum of Weight Problems.

This is important when you want to work with weight problems and resolve, improve or manage them in a better way.

You see; certain aspects of a weight problem are common regardless of what type of weight problem you have. Whether this is someone being too fat or too thin.

These common issues include things like Self-Esteem, Self-Perception, Self-Expectations, Confidence, Motivation and general Unhappiness.

Other aspects of a weight problem are unique to where the weight problem is on the Spectrum of weight problems.

For example: If someone is too fat then they would need to lose weight and someone who is too thin would need to gain weight. Obvious right!

However both the person who is too fat and the person who is too thin can both have a problem with vitamin deficiency and malnourishment. Not so obvious!

The Spectrum of Weight Problems we will be working with, will include the entire Spectrum of weight problems.

At one end of the Spectrum we will be looking at weight problems from the position of those who are very overweight and considered to be Morbidly Obese.

The Morbidly Obese are the very large people who can spend most of their lives in a bed or room because they are too large to move around without assistance. In effect they have become physically disabled by their weight.

At the other end of the Spectrum we will be looking at weight problems from the position of those who are very underweight and who have problems associated with being very underweight. This would include Anorexia.

We will also be looking at weight problems that fall between these two extremes and we will be looking at what is considered to be the Normal Weight Range.

This process of looking across the entire Spectrum of Weight Problems enables us to look at problems that include what we may call "Normal Weight Problems".

And we will be looking at those who are beginning to edge out of the normal weight range and move into the more problematic ranges of weight related problems. This group of people is increasing in number as each year passes.

As well as considering the weight problems themselves, we will also be looking at what leads to persistent weight problems and what sustains weight problems.

Persistent weight problems do not exist in a vacuum and we know that there are issues which contribute to the development of persistent weight problems and to the maintenance and further development of a persistent weight problem.

We also know that weight problems cause or contribute to the development of additional problems. Which can include physical, social, emotional and psychological challenges.

Weight related problems are in fact:

> Life related problems that have the ability to manifest themselves in weight related issues and other associated issues.

Many people who have developed weight problems can also develop problems with alcohol, smoking, relationships, drugs and pretty much any other form of behaviour that can become Over Used or problematic.

There are also many people who will develop problems with alcohol, drugs, sex, violence and the many and varied different problems, difficulties and challenges of Life; but will not have a problem with their weight.

With each person the difficulty is in sorting out the

mess that accumulates over time and which gets distorted by everyday life and Normal Human Dynamics.

The Life mess that people experience tends to fall into the Life areas of:

- Lifestyle
- Wealth
- Health
- Well-being

With each person the Good and the Bad can become confused and intermingled like a Gordian Knot. I would like to attempt to unravel this problematic mix and find a way forwards.

If we take a simplistic approach to dealing with weight related problems, such as is used by most of the weight control programmes in the world, then we actually propagate the myth that we can deal with all weight problems by this simplistic approach.

In reality; by taking this simplistic approach we end up trying to deal with the problem by dealing with a symptom of the problem and not the causes.

The simplistic approach leads on to what I call "Symptom Solutioning©".

Symptom Solutioning leads people to a process of chasing quick fixes and inappropriate and uncapable solutions.

In reality if you have tried to fix something once or

twice using quick fixes and it hasn't worked; then you really should stop wasting your time, money and efforts looking for more of the same.

You need to recognise that there comes a point where you need to stop dealing with the symptom (the persistent weight problem) and begin to deal with the real problem (what is causing and supporting the persistent weight problem).

This can be done by almost everyone; if they have the Will and the tools to do so. I want to help you get the tools; you need to bring or develop the Will.

Within this book and within the scope of what I want to achieve with it. I am recognising that each person will have their own Back Story.

Their Back Story is their own unique mix of things that have taken them to where they are now, and which helps them to stay where they are, and which helps prevent them from achieving what they want from life.

In my experience that Back Story often tends to hold great strengths, which if employed correctly, can help the person out of the shadow of a persistent weight problem and into the sunshine of a better quality of life.

> *It always seemed strange to me that so many diet and exercise experts fail to understand the Back Story of people with weight problems or that there even is a Back Story behind a weight problem.*

In this book I will introduce you to a process that I developed called:

The Dieter's Scale©.

This is a simple and easy process that helps you to begin looking at your weight problem in a different way.

In The Dieters Scale© I use Green, Amber and Red Zones.

These different Zones will help you understand the different ways in which different things can impact your life and affect your weight problem.

Through the use of these Zones, we can begin to understand the real shape of your weight problem and the real shape of the solution that you need to improve and change your life.

The Dieter's Scale© will prepare you for the Human Dynamics Matrix© which I will introduce you to at the end of the book.

> A way to understand this is that The Dieters Scale© gives us the overall shape of things; and the Human Dynamics Matrix lets us fill in the details.

Please do not be afraid of the Human Dynamics Matrix© as it is a very useful tool that I developed to help me work with and understand complicated problems; such as persistent weight problems.

The Dieters Scale© will help you to better understand why and how many of the things that you have tried in the past have not worked, will not work or could not have worked.

It will also help you to see and understand how you need to do things, so that they can and will work to help you effectively deal with a long term weight problem and the Back Story that goes with your individual weight problem.

In this book I will be looking at the best and most effective diet in the world and seeing how you can use this to help you with your weight problem.

This is not going to be what you are used too or what you expect!

I also have an unusual approach to diet structures.

I will not give you a strict diet to follow or say that you cannot eat this or that.

I will make suggestions about your dietary practices that I know have helped people in the past and that still will do so today.

We will look at different things; such as the role of exercise and how I think many people would be better off approaching exercise in a different way.

I will also look at the other ways of measuring your weight that I think are often much more productive than constantly looking at your weight on a scale.

Throughout this book I will be looking to help you better understand what a weight related problem is.

And then we will look at how to improve, resolve or better manage weight related problems; so that we can have a positive influence on a weight problem.

Overall; I will see if I can help you to adjust your perceptions, understandings and thinking around weight related problems and help you to become a more successful person.

A Person who is:

> Living a life without dieting pressures and disappointments.

DON'T JUST READ THIS BOOK ONCE.

KEEP IT HANDY SO THAT YOU CAN REFER TO IT WHEN YOU NEED TO.

CHAPTER 2

Imperfect People!

In this book and others I use the phrase:

Imperfect People

So who or what do I mean by Imperfect People?

When we are dealing with an issue such as a weight problem; Image, Self-Perceptions and our Comparative Perceptions are very important.

It doesn't matter whether we are being accurate or not with Our Perceptions and Our Understanding of things. The reality is that we have the ones that we have; whether they are serving us well or serving us badly.

We are where we are with things and this is what we have to deal with; Our Reality!

And Our Reality is "The Problem" for most people.

On the one side you have the persistent weight problem. And on the other you have the Life Realities that we find difficult to deal with; and that we may not understand; and that we cannot really cope with.

And in the middle of this; there is You!

If we are not prepared, willing or able to deal with Our Own Reality. Then how can we really deal with a weight problem that is part of that reality or which comes out of that reality?

I created "The Imperfect People" concept to help people to better understand and deal with the impact that our perceptions, our understandings and our misunderstanding of things has upon our Lives and the things that we do.

It is designed to help you when you are stuck in the middle between the persistent weight problem and the Life problems.

It's a way of being able to understand and deal with things without having to beat yourself up or feel bad.

When things go wrong: Instead of desperately trying to find answers, or blaming yourself and beating yourself up; why not try something else?

Try allowing yourself to be:

An Imperfect Person.

You see the reality is:

THAT NO-ONE IS PERFECT!

Over the years I have met and talked with many very attractive and beautiful women. From models, to high profile singers, to royalty and those very lovely and beautiful women who populate everyday life.

Being a man I am interested in women but I have also met men who are the same mix.

Very attractive and very handsome men from all walks of life; high profile performers, politicians, academics and people from wealthy and privileged backgrounds, as well as self-made millionaires.

In every person there are flaws. Some of which are real and many which exist just in the mind of the person themselves.

However; the ability to Compare Apples and Pears and see Peaches, is part of the make-up of every person.

As a result, when we see someone who is slim and attractive and we feel overweight and unattractive; are we concerned when the slim attractive person says that they don't like their smile?

Or do we find ourselves saying something like:

> What have they got to complain about! With a figure like that and looks like that; I wish that I had problems like that. Now if they had my...

I am sure that you can fill in the rest of that?

How often have I heard people with weight problems say things like:

- If only I was taller.
- I am big boned.
- Its genetic.
- I have a slow metabolism.
- I only have to look at food to put on weight.
- It's my allergies.
- It's my medication.
- If only I could get sick and stop eating; think how much weight I could lose.
- Some people stop eating when they get upset, I wish I could; all I do is eat.
- I don't have time to eat properly.

And so on and so on. I am sure that you could add to this list?

Another thing that happens to people with weight problems is the Perception Distortions they will experience.

Let me explain.

How often have you heard people say things like:

> If only I could... Then I am sure that I would be able to sort out my weight problem as I would feel so much better and able to do it.

And if they do manage to sort out... How often do they then continue to the next stage of actually sorting out the other problem?

In reality it is often the case that when they do feel better, it leads them to the conclusion that; perhaps things weren't as bad as they thought they really were.

And they do nothing.

And the window of opportunity closes; and they find themselves back in the problem.

How often has this happened to you or someone you know?

Another thing that we do is that we have the ability to see and focus on that which we are worried about or self-conscious off.

Let me explain.

When you are looking at yourself in a mirror or you happen to catch your reflection in a window; what do you notice?

Do you notice that spot on your face or do you see a great looking person and think how great they look?

- Are you noticing with a Critical Negative View or with a Critical Positive View?

The point I am making is that Other People seem as if they are perfect or are capable of being perfect people; but the reality is that we are all Other People to someone.

When we make the Comparison to ourselves and our situation, Other People may seem as if they have perfect lives or that they are perfect people.

But in reality there is no such thing as the Perfect Person. They don't exist!

So this means that we are all Imperfect People.

Because we are Imperfect People we can give ourselves a break, cut ourselves some slack, take the pressure off ourselves: And begin the process of achieving the Life we really would like to be living and experiencing.

In my experience many people have the Desire and Wish to be rid of their persistent weight problem and the difficulties which it creates for them.

However; many, many people are not in a position where they really understand:

- What they need to do?
- How they need to do it?
- Why they need to do it?
- When they need to do it?
- And the Effects and Affects that they are going to go through to achieve a real sustainable positive result.

The answer to this question is one of the things which determines the outcome of people efforts:

> Are they Willing, Able and Prepared to do what is required to finally deal with this problem?

There is another aspect to this that many people shy away from or try to ignore.

Personally I think that this is a key to success for many people with persistent weight problems.

When we are dealing with a persistent weight problem we have to accept:

The Reality of Failure.

In my experience Failure is part of the Reality of Successfully dealing with difficult problems that involve Weight.

It might seem strange to you to think that Failure with your weight problem is a good thing; but it is if it is dealt with in the right way.

You see a weight problem becomes entangled with your life and how you live and manage your life.

When something goes wrong with your Life, then it will affect your weight problem.

It is at times of crisis, difficulty and hardship that people fail with diets.

It is also at times of great joy and happiness that people fail with diets.

It is also when anniversaries come around each year and someone remembers something or someone; that people fail with diets.

And it is also true that when things are going really well and someone is achieving all the things that they want; that people fail with diets.

The reality is that failure is part of the process of success and we will deal with that later on in this book.

Another very important thing is that when it comes to weight issues we can have very limited viewpoints on certain subjects.

We can suffer from:

- Selective Hearing.
- Selective Seeing.
- Selective Understanding.
- Selective Insights.
- Selective Self-Perceptions; just to name a few!

Another thing that we can do, as Imperfect People, is to Compare Apple and Pears and see Peaches.

This means that we can use our Insecurities; our Self-Doubts; our Attempts at Understanding Ourselves and our Desire Not To Be as We Are:

> We can use these things to convince ourselves of many different things which we know, hope or fear could be true.

This makes us Vulnerable!

It makes us vulnerable at many different levels and some people will realise the extent of their vulnerability and others will not.

For many; their ability to convince themselves of whatever they want to believe:

> Will be being used to fuel Negative Self-Perceptions and Negative and Destructive Behaviour.

All of this stuff is all part of the Back Story of different people. And all this stuff may seem gloomy and difficult and even impossible to deal with.

The reality is different!

> All of this stuff has the seeds of great outcomes buried inside of it.

You see this stuff can be turned around and focused on Positive things rather than Negative things.

If you actually realised the amount of effort, time and resources that it takes to have an unsatisfactory life; you would be surprised.

What I am interested in is changing the focus of all that negative stuff and making it work for you; rather than against you.

So what do I want you to take away from this chapter?

It is this:

I'm an Imperfect Person;

And I have the ability to improve;

And I have the ability to have a better life;

And Being an Imperfect Person;

Is OK!

CHAPTER 3

Where Are You On The Dieters Scale?

I want you to begin to get an idea of the structure of your persistent weight problem.

We are going to achieve this by using The Dieters Scale ©.

The Dieters Scale© has 3 different Zones. These are coloured Green, Amber and Red.

The different problems, difficulties and challenges that we all face in life, will tend to be located in one or more of these 3 Zones.

By answering a few simple questions we can begin to see and understand how your weight problem is structured.

So what we are going to do is to look at 6 questions and then put the answers in the appropriate Zone in The Dieters Scale.

That means that you will end up with answers that will be in either the: Green Zone, Amber Zone or Red Zone.

Some of you may find that your answers don't fit in just one Zone. This is fine.

Question 1

Most people would know, or easily be able to find out, what is considered to be their right weight, given their physical build, age and other relevant factors.

Now you might not agree with this weight, so if you don't then let's do this:

Find out what that weight is and then make a note of it. Then work out what you consider to be the right weight for you and then write down what you consider to be the right weight.

Now if there is more than 1 stone or 7 kilo's difference, between the figure that you prefer and the weight that is considered normal for you; write down; Why you believe your figure is correct and the other one is wrong?

Once you have done this, keep this, and you can refer back to it at another time.

Either way, we should now have a weight that you believe is the right weight for you.

So the next thing we need to know is:

What is your actual weight now?

There is no point cheating with this as I am not going to see the information. You don't have to hide it, be ashamed of it, worried about it or afraid of it.

The truth is that this just gives us a starting point and if you can't NOT cheat at this stage then it tells me something.

What we want this Accurate Information for is to help us place you in the right position in The Dieters Scale©.

> *If you were taking part in one of my Problem Mastery Programmes focused on Weight, then this would be one of the few times that you would be physically weighed.*

In the following graphic you will see that we have 3 sections and they are marked Green, Amber and Red. Underneath each of these colours is a weight.

If your actual weight is different to that Considered to be Your Right Weight; then select which colour corresponds to the difference between the two.

Green	Amber	Red
1 stone (7 Kilo's)	3 stone (22 Kilo's)	More

RAG Testing ©

So: If there is 1 stone difference between your ideal weight and your actual weight; choose Green.

If there is between 1 and 3 stone difference between your ideal weight and your actual weight; then choose Amber.

If there is more than 3 stone difference between your ideal weight and your actual weight; then choose Red.

For those of you who are underweight we will use the same process.

So: If you are 1 stone underweight choose Green.

If you are between 1 and 3 stone underweight then choose Amber.

And if you are more than 3 stone underweight then choose Red.

So write down what your answer was for this:

Green, Amber or Red?

Now we will look at Frequency of Dieting.

Question 2

What I am interested in here is Your Dieting History and how often you will have dieted.

Some people will begin their Dieting History early in their lives and others will begin it later in life.

Generally speaking the older you are, the longer Your Dieting History is likely to be.

The longer Your Dieting History is, the more diets you are likely to have been on.

The more diets you will have been on; then the more of your life that will have been spent dieting.

We will use The Dieters Scale to see where you are with Your Dieting History.

Green	Amber	Red
2 Diets or less	4 Diets or more!	Always Dieting

RAG Testing ©

If you have been on or followed 2 diets or less in your life, then you will be in the Green Zone.

If you have been on or followed 4 diets or more in your life then you will be in the Amber Zone.

If you are always on one diet or another AND you have been on more than 4 dieting episodes, then you will be in the Red Zone.

Now some of you might try and cheat on this one and say that you have been on something like "The No Food Diet" all your life; but the reality is that you know what I mean and you know what the truth of the matter is.

So write down what your answer was for this:

Green, Amber or Red?

Question 3

Now we will look at your ability to stick to a diet and to achieve the desired weight that you want; through that dieting process.

What we want to know is: Have you ever done it?

Have you been able to stick to diets and achieve the desired outcome with your weight?

Green	Amber	Red
Easily stick to diet	Keep to it at bit	No Chance!

RAG Testing ©

If the answer is that you have easily been able to follow and stick to the diet, without cheating, and you stuck with it and achieved the result you wanted:

Then you should choose the Green Zone.

If the answer is that you have started diets with all the best intentions:

- But your struggled.
- You found it difficult.
- You cheated a lot and you got fed-up and bored.
- But you did manage to lose weight and you did feel better being on the diet:

Then you should choose the Amber Zone.

If the answer is that you look at diets and you think that they are great. But when you start them:

- You just can't be bothered.
- Immediately want to eat all the food that is forbidden to you.
- Find that you have no motivation for this; even though it was your idea:

Then you should choose the Red Zone.

Some of you might be carefully reading the text at this point and seeing if you can place yourself in the Zone below where you really should be.

The reality is that you are where you are. The only person that you are going to try and fool here is yourself.

And as you are an expert on you; then it won't really work.

So put down the right Zone!

Question 4

Next we will look at Exercise and the role that exercise has in your daily life and how it influences your weight.

As part of being Human we need to move and do things with our bodies.

We need to use energy to exercise; but to the body exercise is work. As a result the body will be very efficient with the energy that it uses, to do the work that it needs to do.

- The reality is that Exercise is not a very good weight management tool or weight loss method.

Exercise is about maintaining the bodies abilities to perform certain task and to function well.

If we fail to maintain the bodies abilities then we experience consequences.

Those consequences can be short term; as in being generally unfit, a lack of energy, poor sleep, tiredness, poor digestion, etc.

Or; they can be medium and long term consequences such as poor posture, skeletal problems, cardiovascular problems, sleep problems, poor balance and co-ordination, etc.

I personally like to think of exercise as an investment in my life which gives me immediate and long term benefits.

So let's see where you are in your life with this, on the Dieters Scale.

Green	Amber	Red
I am fit! Exercise	Occasional Exercise	Don't!

RAG Testing ©

So: If you are fit and you exercise regularly then you should select the Green Zone.

Regular exercise would be about 3 hours a week (up to about 6 hours) of planned and reasonably demanding periods of exercise, where you break a sweat doing it.

This will be a part of your normal everyday life and you will be maintaining this ongoingly and you will have done so for some time (Months or years).

If you fall into the occasional exercise zone then you should select Amber.

If you occasionally exercise then you won't have a regular weekly programme that you have followed for a long time; or for a reasonable period of time, of say 6 months or more.

Occasional Exercisers may exercise when they feel particularly out of shape or when they are following another diet programme.

They may do things like have the occasional swim or walk. *Please note that going to the swimming pool is not the same as having a good swim.*

The Red zone is for those who know that they are unfit and don't care about it; or who will get around to it one day.

These are the people who would love to take a pill to be fit or if they could get someone else to do it for them, they would.

They know all the arguments for getting fit and they have been told to get fit by their doctors; but they really can't be bothered yet.

On the other hand; they could be people who just don't know about and understand the real benefits of exercise and keeping fit. They may just be uneducated about this area of life and have never engaged with this before.

So are you a Red Zone person?

> Some people are very active but overweight; and some people are underactive and slim.
>
> You should not confuse being overweight with being unfit and you should not confuse being slim with being fit.

Question 5

The next thing we will look at is Stress!

Stress comes in all shapes and sizes; just like people do.

What one person finds stressful another might find to be a challenge. Life is just funny like that!

So what we are interested in is the total level of stress in your life, regardless of where that stress comes from or originates from.

Now stress is a funny thing in many ways. Stress is something which we can Self-Report on and it is something which others can Inform Us Of.

The Self-Reported stress is the stress which we ourselves are aware of and which we respond to. It might be working long hours, putting up with things we don't want to, not getting the things we want out of life, etc.

Generally, Self-Reported Stress is the stress that we are aware off and which we may want to keep private; it can also be the stuff that we talk about to our best friends and try to cope with ourselves.

"The Inform Us Of" stress is when other people notice that we are stressed and they tell us about it.

Often this can be that someone is "Snappy" with other people; when someone is drinking or smoking too much; or when someone is constantly eating.

These are often talked about as "Stress Indicators".

To keep things simple we will bring all the different stresses that you experience together for this exercise.

Green	Amber	Red
No Stress!	Quite Stressed!	Always Stressed

RAG Testing ©

So: if you have no Self-Reported stress and no Inform Us Of stress then you would be in the Green Zone.

If you have the occasional thing which stresses you out but you are not normally stressed by very much; then you would be in the Green Zone.

The Amber Zone is for those people who are quite stressed with life. You will be doing things like:

- Eating far too much; even for you.
- Drinking too much alcohol.
- Taking medication to cope.
- Having more arguments than normal.
- Having trouble sleeping.
- Feeling tired all the time and unable to relax.
- Frequently feeling dissatisfied with your life.

The Red Zone is for those people who are stressed all the time.

You will know that you are in the Red Zone because you won't know what it's like to really relax and be enjoying life.

So which Zone are you in: Green, Amber or Red?

Question 6

The next thing we are going to put into The Dieters Scale is the Negative Experiences that cause us to feel bad about ourselves and to develop Negative Habits.

This includes:

Being Negative; Putting Yourself Down; Negative Self-Talk ; Other People Putting You Down; and Other People Being Negative Towards You.

What we are interested in is the Quality and the Quantity of the Negative Experiences you have on a daily or regular basis.

For example: Something small could have a big impact on you; but you feel that other people might find it small and insignificant. It's is your view of this that matters and not other peoples.

Another example: You may have a friend who turns on you when you are doing well and they begin to undermine you until you get back to the position where they are the one who is on top. This gives you lots of Negative Feedback which amounts to a high Quality and high Quantity Negative Feedback.

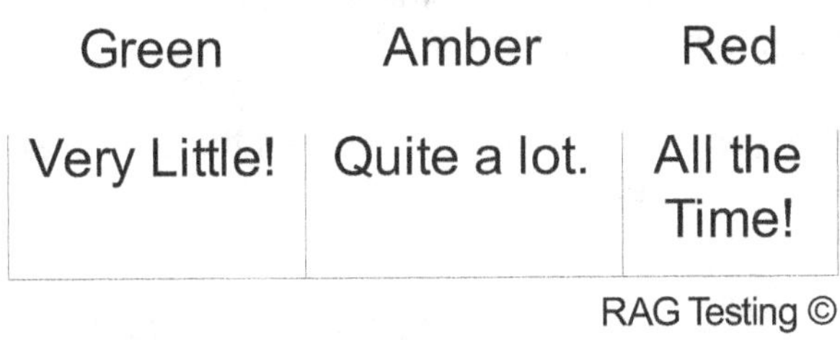

Green	Amber	Red
Very Little!	Quite a lot.	All the Time!

RAG Testing ©

So: If you have very small amounts of Negative Experiences or Negative Self-Talk; then you would be in the Green Zone.

If you experience quite a lot of Negative Experiences or Negative Self-Talk; then you would be in the Amber Zone.

If you have quite a lot of Negative Interactions with other people; then you would be in the Amber Zone.

If you experience a continuous process of Negative Experiences, Feedback or Negative Self-Talk; then you would be in the Red Zone.

If you have a continuous process of Negative Interactions with other people; then you would be in the Red Zone.

So which Zone are you in: Green, Amber or Red?

We could continue to take different life aspects and use the same process to create a larger Dieter's Scale© and build a bigger more informed picture.

However; We will stop at the 6 that we have and see what that is telling us.

In the graphic below I have brought the 6 different questions together.

Green	Amber	Red
1 stone (7 Kilo's)	3 stone (22 Kilo's)	More
2 Diets or less	4 Diets or more!	Always Dieting
Easily stick to diet	Keep to it at bit	No Chance!
I am fit! Exercise	Occasional Exercise	Don't!
No Stress!	Quite Stressed!	Always Stressed
Very Little!	Quite a lot.	All the Time!

RAG Testing ©

If you were to tick the relevant boxes in the Dieters Scale© above, what would this show?

Do you have a mix of all three zones?

Are all your ticks in one zone?

Are your ticks in two zones?

What I would expect you to see is the following:

If you are OVERWEIGHT with a long dieting history, then your ticks should be predominantly in the Amber and Red Zones.

If you are UNDERWEIGHT with a long dieting history, then your ticks should be predominantly in the Amber and Red Zones.

If you are between the two extremes of being very underweight and being very overweight, then I would expect that you would have a mixture of two or all three Zones.

If I added more questions to The Dieters Scale© we could bring in more elements of the Weight and the Weight Related problems to increase the general overview.

Personally; I find that the Dieters Scale is a useful tool that can provide us with information that can be helpful.

Looking at and understanding what we need to be working with, by breaking it down into Zones; makes the problem less formidable.

Working with The Dieters Scale© is also a good way to work towards using the Human Dynamics Matrix©.

The Human Dynamics Matrix helps me to see the problem in a different way and it helps me to understand and work with the Back Story that everyone has.

> The Human Dynamics Matrix helps me get under the skin of the problem and begin to see the actual skeletal shape of that structure.

So what do I want you to take away from this chapter?

We have looked at the Dieters Scale and seen that we have 3 Zones. Green, Amber and Red.

You have completed 6 simple questions and it provided a brief and simple indicator of where you were in those Zones.

Dependent to your answers. You may have been in 1 Zone or all 3 of them.

If you have a persistent weight problem then you will have tried different diets and probably been to organised classes for weight control. So let me ask you to think about this:

> You now know that we can put peoples weight problems into one of 3 Zones.
>
> So when we see people from the Green Zone in a diet class with people from the Amber and Red Zones; and they are all applying the same solution to their problem; is it any wonder that the long term success rate is very low?

In many cases I think that the Problem Mix that someone with a persistent weight problem has, is beyond the capacity of the solution that they are using to try and fix it.

This is why we have a growing problem with weight and weight related issues. Too often it's a case of square pegs and round holes. They simply just don't go together!

CHAPTER 4

The Most Successful Diet In The World!

What is the most successful and the best diet in the world?

The reality is: That it depends!

> What is it that you want to achieve from the diet; both in the short term and in the long term?
>
> Do you want to keep going on diets or do you want to get yourself on the right path for a successful life in the future?

Being someone who designs solutions for problems; I thought that a much better way to approach this question was to actually design the most successful and best diet in the world; for every person.

I am not interested in designing bad solutions. So I want to design:

A Great World Class Solution.

So let's create the Most Successful and the Best Diet in the World; that will get you on the right path and be able to keep you there!

Let's begin with a simple question.

> If we were to design the most successful and the best diet in the world, **for any person**; what would it look like?

And this is what I came up with:

The best diet in the world is one that fits into your lifestyle today and into the lifestyle that you want to have in the future; without undue pressure and demands.

The best diet in the world isn't bothered by the occasional dietary indiscretion; because it allows for it to happen.

The best diet in the world is one that you can stick too; without undue pressure and without feeling that you are being deprived of the things that you like.

The best diet in the world is the one that helps you achieve the weight control that you really want to achieve; and be able to help you maintain it over the longer term.

The best diet in the world is personal to you.

The best diet in the world is not temperamental, it is robust, strong and full of vitality for you to share.

The best diet in the world is easy to follow and does not have a rigid structure that you have to slavishly follow.

It does not rely exclusively upon points, calorie counting and having a very limited diet.

The best diet in the world does not make false claims about weight loss and play tricks with your body.

The best diet in the world knows that you want to live for a long time and have a high quality of life; for the rest of your life.

The best diet in the world helps you to understand and work with your own Personal Tendencies; so that you can achieve and maintain the life that you want.

The best diet in the world does not ban any foods; but it does require moderation at times and that you take responsibility for what you consume.

The best diet in the world recognises that you are an Imperfect Person and accepts that you will have to learn and adapt; and that occasionally, you will make mistakes that you will both have to put right.

The best diet in the world will become like a brother, sister or best friend; always there to help and support you for the rest of your life.

The best diet in the world wants to become your new best friend, but you have to make a decision about how much time, effort and money you are willing to put into developing and maintaining that friendship.

The best diet in the world is something that you Do. Not something that you talk about doing.

The best diet in the world doesn't expect you to be a Perfect Person and achieve quick lasting results.

It knows that you are not Perfect and it wants to have a lifelong relationship with you.

The best diet in the world recognises its own limitations and that it does not exist in isolation to the other parts of your life that touch and are touched by food and by eating habits.

Do you want the best and most successful diet in the world?

In reality the best and the most successful diet in the world is made up of different components which can be adapted individually for each person.

There are no rigid time restraints and it is a mistake to apply any.

No part of it is too difficult or over demanding of you, your abilities or your lifestyle.

Nor are there any demands for you to lose or gain weight quickly.

There are no ongoing measurements saying things like; this week you must lose (X) amount of weight; this week you should be so many inches slimmer when we measure various points of your body; or that you must drop a dress size; or any other pressure point.

There is Reality which is grounded in the reality of your lifestyle; and the Reality of the different aspects of your life, behaviour, habits, psychology and emotional responses.

There are challenges and expectations that are part of the process of having and using the best diet in the world. That is because you want to achieve something and you want to improve, resolve and better manage different aspects of your life.

The best and most successful diet in the world is about mutual co-operation between you; the diet and the lifestyle management process you are using.

The best and most successful diet in the World is about:

- Doing things when the time is right.
- In the right way.
- And with the correct application of actions.

All of this is what I do when I am working with someone on a Problem Mastery Programme; where Weight is the focus of the Programme.

> Different Components of "The Most Successful and Best Diet In the World" come into play at different times.
>
> As the Dynamics of the Person and their Individual Circumstances, and Problem Mix require it.

It is Usual that the person I am working with does NOT see the full picture of what is happening at the time. And it is with Hindsight that they begin to appreciate the work that we have been doing and the progress that they have made.

Another important aspect of successfully dealing with long term persistent weight problems is Time.

Many of the different components have their own time scale and conditions that cannot be shortened.

If you try to shorten them, then what happens is that you cannot deal with them properly and you end up having to deal with a consequence. Then the problems can come back again.

In my opinion and experience Real Success with Weight is NOT achieved by someone following a diet or exercise plan that claims they could lose 14 pounds (6kg) in 14 days and get fit in 6 weeks (or variations of this).

Nor is it achieved by Diet Pills or Surgery which limits someone's ability to Consume More or which limits the effects of increased consumption.

They don't work because:

Quick and simple solutions to complicated and difficult problems rarely work well.

Normally, in my view, the simple diet and exercise approaches can work best for those who would be all Green on our Dieters Scale.

People who are in the Green Zone not just for our 6 questions but for additional ones as well.

These are the people who have a small to moderate weight problem; and if they focus just on the weight problem then they can change it.

However; they may not be able to maintain the weight loss and this should be viewed as an indicator that other factors are in play and influencing the problem. And that their weight problem is not as Green as they believe it is.

Those who have Amber Zone and Red Zone problems will usually fail with the simple diet and exercise approaches.

They will need the Best and Most Effective Diet in the World to succeed.

So what do I want you to take away from this chapter?

A weight management process which majors on food, food consumption and the provision of food products to its customers; may well have a conflict of interest in the ethical framework of its business model.

The ethical framework aside.

The simple reality, in my view, is that the process that focuses on food is doomed to failure for most of the people who use the process; because the process can only give them a part of what they really need.

In the short term it can satisfy their need to feel as if they are doing something and taking charge of the problem. But the tools that they are using are inadequate for the task they really need to perform.

A persistent weight problem is about more than food for most people and dealing with this successfully requires a different structure to the one that a diet brings.

Those who fall into the Amber and Red sections of the Dieters Scale© will usually find that they will really struggle, and continue to fail, when they follow these food focused weight control plans.

One way to look at a weight problem is:

> That part of your life is telling you that it is time to change what and how you are living.
>
> Because what you are doing, and how you are doing it, is not giving you what you really want and what you really need.
>
> In effect:
>
> The persistent weight problem becomes a Life Barometer.

CHAPTER 5

Eat What You Want; Just Accept The Consequences!

When I work with people who have problems with their weight; they usually expect me to provide them with a diet sheet, weigh them and tell them all the things that they can no longer do.

I don't do that because by the time I normally see people, they have already been through the weight loss process a number of times.

By the time they get to me I find that they have a lot of experience with diets, and all that goes with dieting.

They have a lot of Experience about what they will actually do and what they won't actually do.

And this is what I really want to work with:

- The Experience that They Are Aware of.
- And the Experience that They Are Unaware of.

What I am interested in is helping someone to change their weight problem; by working with and changing the structure that supports and maintains their weight problem.

As part of doing this; I am looking for common patterns of behaviour. And for things which are there but which people tend not to see or understand.

With weight related problems there is a Human Dynamic which I see repeatedly.

> A Human Dynamic is a process, structure or behaviour; which has a consistent form or pattern to it, that involves or relates to people.
>
> So it is something that people do often; in a predictable way.

The Human Dynamic I am referring to is:

> Someone has a problem and they want to do something about that problem.
>
> What is Motivating them to do so is that they don't like the Consequences that the problem is producing and how it is Affecting things.
>
> What they continually attempt to do is to apply a solution but only to that part of the problem that is most bothering them.
>
> While doing this they try to leave other things as they are; by not dealing with any other associated problem or issue.
>
> They don't want to rock-the-boat in case it upsets too many things in their lives and they won't be able to handle it.

So they find themselves in the position where they want changes to occur; but just with the single problem they are focused on and nothing else.

They often feel that if they can deal with their single problem, that they will then be able to better cope with all the other stuff that is going on around them.

Sometimes people manage this trick but most of the time they don't.

They might get a brief respite from the problem but it usually doesn't last.

What can also happen with this approach is that the problem itself and the related problems; actually become worse.

In effect; what happens is that this "I will go on a diet" approach to problem solving; becomes part of the persons Coping Mechanisms and Life Strategies.

The adoption of this problem solving strategy occurs because it partly works for a period of time. Because it partly works it continues to be used.

Eventually however it fails. But in the process we can end up with the habits of the classic Yo-Yo Dieter being created by this process.

This Human Dynamic is, in effect, the Human Dynamic which underpins many dieting approaches.

> Deal with the obvious problem (their weight) and hope that it creates enough momentum to improve other things as well (all the other problems).
>
> Their weight is also the easiest common factor to focus on and use to market to those with weight problems.

The tragedy of this approach is that there is a time in the development of a problem when you can apply a solution that will work.

If you wait and don't apply the solution; then the window of opportunity closes and the structure of the problem changes.

Once the structure of the problem changes; the structure of the solution also needs to change.

As it is with this Human Dynamic so it is with weight related problems.

> The nature of the weight problem changes as you move from one Zone to another Zone; and so the nature of the solution that the problem requires; also changes.

The same is true of any problem. For example:

> If you drink alcohol and you have an alcohol problem which is in the Green Zone, it will

> require a different solution to the alcohol problem being experienced by the person who has a problem which is in the Amber or Red Zones.

What complicates things for most people is that problems develop, and as they develop they connect with other things that can also become problems.

> As problems developed they tend not to go in a straight line; it is more like the creation of a spiders web.

This means that by the time something becomes a big enough issue for someone to want to sort out, it touches, influences and is influenced by other things as well.

So you end up in a position where you don't just have one thing which needs sorting out; you have multiple things.

I call this a Basket of Problems.

For most people dealing with a Basket of Problems becomes overwhelming!

They don't know where to start, how to do it or what they should be doing.

This is when it becomes easier to deal with the obvious problem and hope that it has a knock-on effect with the other problems.

> This is a Human Algorithm at work.

Because we are all Imperfect People we will look for easy solutions if we can find them.

> However: Easy doesn't mean Effective!

When I work with people and we look at the Basket of Problems that someone has, it is not uncommon to find that one part of the problem mix is in the Green Zone, another part of the problem mix is in the Amber Zone and another part of the problem mix is in the Red Zone.

> Ok; dealing with this can be complicated and difficult; but you have to remember that we are dealing with this over time and in a planned way.

So let's focus this back on to the subject of this chapter.

Eat what you want; just accept the consequences.

To deal with weight problems effectively:

> People need to accept that it is they who are experiencing the problem;
>
> Therefore, they are part of the problem;
>
> Therefore, they need to be part of the solution;
>
> Therefore, they need to be Pro-Active in achieving the results that they want:

Because if they wait on other people to do it for them:

> They will be caught in the Human Dynamic that we have been looking at; and things will have a Tendency to become worse, rather than better.

So to achieve what they want; they need to begin to be Pro-Active!

Being Pro-Active means taking Positive Actions to deal with something. Rather than waiting for things to happen to you; and then responding to events by reacting to them. I.e. Being Re-Active.

It is the practice of Being Pro-Active that is behind:

Eat what you want; just accept the consequences.

In a later chapter I will take you through a breakdown of the different things that are going on when someone goes on a diet.

Amongst those things are an increase in stress, the removal of coping strategies and the introduction of new behaviours.

So there are plenty of new and different things going on for the person; and we know that they are going to have difficulties dealing with it all.

My view was that rather than do what other people are doing with weight problems; why not do something different?

So I said to myself:

- So why not give them back some Control?
- Why not give them back some Choices?
- Why not use this process to help them understand Their Own Behaviour?
- Why not use all the Experience that they have?
- Why not take away some of the Stress?

So I took the approach that I would not give them a diet plan.

I would not tell them to exercise.

I would not tell them that they could NOT eat certain foods.

There were a number of other things as well but I will not go into those here.

All that I asked them to do was to accept that if they eat any food, that they accepted the potential disappointments and consequences of their actions.

I gave them the Freedom to make their own decisions and the Permission that they were free to eat what they chose to eat.

> Why pretend that you love “healthy food” when all you want to do is eat burger and chips?

The reality that I am accepting here is that by the time I am seeing people; their metabolism’s are messed up.

> Their eating habits are all over the place and their bodies have lost reference to the Normal that they are attempting to achieve through dieting.

So if we do what is normally done through the dieting process; our chances of success are actually low.

By changing the approach that we take; we actually increase our chances of a successful outcome.

Our chances of Success are higher!

Within this process I am accepting a truth that I have seen many times:

> It can actually be months before the person brings themselves to the point where we have a diet structure in place that they Can and Will follow.

It doesn't matter that it takes this long because when we get there, we are in a very strong position and we begin to work on and build on a different foundation. A foundation that can support the work we need to do.

As we go through this process it ceases to be about Weight control and it begins to be about Life Improvement, Development and Management.

So Weight becomes just one of the components of a Life Improvement Programme and the importance of it reduces over time.

This is the Smart Way!

So what do I want you to take away from this chapter?

If you have a weight problem, then you are the arena where the problem is going to be played out.

As you are the arena then you can exercise control over different things.

> What you consume is one of those things over which you can exercise control.
>
> When you do exercise control; just accept that whatever the consequences are; you will accept them.
>
> Your decisions and choices will have an effect which is Positive or Negative.

You can deal with your persistent weight problem in the way that the problem requires you to; or you can just keep doing the same things and hope that you get lucky.

The problem with luck is that you can't rely on it and when you need it; it is seldom around.

Dealing with the problem as it requires you to; is the Smart Way to do so.

You waste less time, less effort and the disappointments you avoid are huge.

Chapter 6

Food Addiction - Fact Or Myth?

I can see the attraction of having Food Addiction as an explanation for many of the weight problems that people have.

I can also see that there would be a dramatic increase in the number of people who would claim that it is not their fault that they have a weight problem; because they are Addicted to food.

Would this be a good thing?

As a result of this approach it would not be long before their persistent weight problem would become a Medical Condition.

> The reality is that many people are trying to find the so called “Fat Gene”. And because of the consequences of Obesity; Obesity has become a medicalised condition.

As a medical condition there would be the view that there must be a medical remedy to fix this Medical Problem.

I can see that the preference for the medical remedy would be in the form of a pill, or procedure, which quickly and simply cures them of their weight problem.

And once the remedy is applied; the view of many would be that they should never have another problem with their weight, regardless of their eating habits, because they have been cured of that problem!

Once we have Food Addiction as an acceptable Claim, it would not be long before people would begin to blame food for their other Life problems and the difficulties in Life that they experience.

They will take less and less personal responsibility for their own actions and the consequences of those actions.

By this process they will also Disempower themselves.

> Would you really want to be Disempowered further?

You see if eating and losing control of your weight, really is something that you cannot control. And if it is true that you are suffering from a medical complaint.

Then really you are not in a position to be able to make any form of Informed Decision about your treatment; as you can't exercise any control over it.

This seems to leave you in the position where Doctors and Politicians would have to determine your treatment.

This would have to be regardless of your wishes because you are, according to your own pronounced views, powerless in the face of this condition and unable to control what you do.

The pertinent questions for this chapter are:

> Is Food Addiction real?
>
> Will the label of "Food Addict" help or hinder someone's attempts at dealing with a weight problem; in the short and long term?

I will give you my take on this and we will see what it produces.

What I am going to do is to break the Food Addiction question down into sections and go through them.

Let's begin with Physical Addiction to a substance.

We will begin with this because simply put:

> If there is No physical addiction to a specifically identifiable substance, as a result of the consumption and/or use of the substance; then there is No Addiction.

You might find some of this difficult to understand but you can always come back to it later and read it in sections.

I will make this a simple as it can be while still covering the relevant points.

Physical Substance Addiction

To understand Physical Substance Addiction, I am going to use the categories of Drugs and Alcohol to illustrate the processes involved.

> Food Addiction would follow the same processes as addiction to drugs and alcohol; as we are talking about the Consumption and Use of a Substance by the body, to which it becomes directly or indirectly physically addicted.

Just about everyone is familiar with and has had exposure to Drugs and Alcohol, so you should be able to follow me.

Drugs includes prescription drugs, as prescription drugs can be as addictive and be misused in the same way as illicit and unlawful drug taking.

I am going to break the addiction problem down into 2 inter-related areas:

1. Their Physical Exposure to Drugs and Alcohol – *The actual Consumption and physiological effects/affects produced.*

2. Their Psycho-Social Exposure to Drugs and Alcohol – *Also called Socialising.*

As our starting point: Let's begin with a person who has never used, taken or consumed Drugs or Alcohol of any type in their lives before.

This person would be a Drugs and Alcohol Virgin.

> Therefore their Physical Exposure to Drugs and Alcohol is Zero!

As well as never having Physically taken drugs or alcohol. We will also say that they will have had no Social Exposure to drug and alcohol use.

This means that they will never have come into contact with or been around those who have or who do use them.

> So their Psycho-Social Exposure to Drugs and Alcohol would also be Zero.

Psycho-Social Exposure would also include exposure to marketing, news stories, films, television, as well as stories and experiences about how and why other people use alcohol or drugs as they do.

As a result of this Zero Exposure and Contact; the persons understanding and appreciation of Alcohol and Drugs usage is clean and uncorrupted.

They have; No Influences related to it of any kind.

This means that we could think of them as a new born baby.

> Rather than bounce between drugs and alcohol, I will focus just on alcohol. What we are interested in is the Addiction and this will be the same regardless of the substance that we are considering.

So let's create an Alcohol Drinking History for this person and follow it through.

Let's say that: Initially this person's use of Alcohol is strictly social and they begin using alcohol at 18 years of age.

As they become older their social use of alcohol increases and they begin using Alcohol more frequently.

Throughout this period the person maintains their work, home and social life without problems.

At this early stage there are no Social problems with Alcohol or as a result of their consuming Alcohol.

In the person's body there have been no obvious changes due to the consumption of Alcohol.

So there is no sign of Clinical Addition to a substance.

Gradually, over time, the person increases their consumption of Alcohol and the frequency and amounts increase.

At first it is within the normal range, let's say 18 units of alcohol per week (2 bottles of wine).

More time passes and different life problems occur.

To help them deal with the different aspects of life, which can be both Positive and Negative, the person consumes more alcohol and this increased consumption becomes a daily occurrence.

Their consumption increases from 18 units per week to 40 units, then to 60 units and then to 80 units.

At 80 units they are consuming about 1.3 bottles of wine per day.

And let's say that this increases further to about 100 units per week; which is about 1.5 bottles of wine per day.

Now let's say that this person continues drinking at this level for a reasonable period of time; let's say 5 years for example.

What will have happened over the time that the person has been consuming alcohol at the higher levels is:

> That the person's body will have first become accustomed to the alcohol.
>
> Then: As it becomes accustomed to the alcohol; it builds up a tolerance to it.

The tolerance the body builds up allows the person to consume more without necessarily experiencing increased Effects and Affects from the increasing consumption of alcohol.

> With the consumption of all these Addictive Substances, there is a point at which a line is

crossed; and this line varies from person to person.

As we cross this line, the body adjusts to a State where it is normal for the body to have alcohol in it.

This line is a point at which things can change for the person in a number of different ways.

These Changes can influence all their further usages of alcohol; either directly or indirectly.

Once someone crosses this line; there can be changes within organs, such as the Liver, and different physiological and psychological changes can occur.

Some of the changes can be permanent and some temporary.

Let's move on from having crossed the line!

So now the bodies normal state is that it should have 1.5 bottles of wine each day.

And the body has adjusted in different ways to deal with and process the alcohol that the person is consuming.

If at this point; we now take the alcohol away from the person they will experience problems.

This is because their Body and their Psyche have got used to having 1.5 bottles of wine each day.

For their body, it has become normal to have to handle the wine and the alcohol that the wine contains.

In preparation for the consumption of the wine; the body has prepared itself to deal with the alcohol it receives each day.

In preparation it will adjust the bodies chemistry and processes so as to convert and manage what is contained within the wine.

During the period since the person was 18, there has been a gradual process occurring.

> The person's Body, their Social Habits and Psyche have all adapted to the increased use and consumption of the alcohol and it has become Normal for them.

So if we now Remove Alcohol and stop or greatly reduce its use; what will happen?

By removing the alcohol from the body, we deprive the body of something that it is expecting and which it has prepared itself to handle.

Having 1.5 bottles of wine a day to process has become the Normal Condition. So removal of the wine from the body becomes An Abnormal Act.

The Body has prepared for the alcohol and now wants it.

Without the 1.5 bottles of wine a day, the body will now Protest and produce consequences.

What is happening is that the Body is responding to the removal of the Substance: Alcohol; which it has come to expect as Normal.

> And the persons Psyche and their Social Habits are all out of sorts because alcohol is no longer being consumed.
>
> These also have come to rely upon the use of alcohol and the habits and customs that develop around its use.

So all of these areas: Physical, Social and their Psyche have become entwined with the use and consumption of the alcohol.

> The Psyche and the Social Habits respond due to the Dependency and Reliance that they have built up for "The Role" that Alcohol and Alcohol Related Behaviour performs in their Management and Operation of the person's Life; at both a personal and social level.

This is the evidence of Physical Substance Addiction:

> If the body is given the required amount of alcohol it will stop protesting and return to what has become the New Normal for it.
>
> If it isn't provided with the required amount of alcohol, it will continue to protest until such time as its need for the alcohol abates.
>
> We call this process Withdrawal or Detox.

The Pattern and Process of Withdrawal from alcohol tends to be consistent and predictable.

Once the physical need for the alcohol abates, then the person is no longer Physically Addicted to the substance of alcohol.

Once Withdrawal is completed the body adjusts to the point where it is no longer Normal for it to process 1.5 bottles of wine each day.

The New Normal now becomes that no alcohol is given to the body to process.

As a result the body is now NOT clinically addicted to alcohol any more.

From this point forwards; if the person never consumes alcohol in any form then they will not become addicted to alcohol again.

However; the person will not necessarily be free from the strong desires and impulses to use and consume alcohol.

The strong desires and intense compulsions to consume alcohol will continue; but it is not being driven by the Addiction to alcohol.

It can't be because: The Actual Physical Addiction has now been removed!

Now what remains and can drive the strong desires and intense compulsions to consume alcohol is the Psycho-Social elements.

For our Addiction problem:

> We still have the Psycho-Social elements to address and these are usually far more difficult to deal with than the physical addiction to the substance.

This is because they both supported and have become Dependent upon the use of alcohol; and all the behaviours around alcohol consumption.

Alcohol consumption facilitated the Psycho-Social Elements in doing their job. Take away the Alcohol and they now need to find new ways of doing so.

> We need to understand that the use of alcohol provided structures to the person that helped them deal with and make sense of different things in Life: In addition to those which related directly to alcohol.
>
> This may include things like; managing relationships, how to socialise, coping with stress at home and at work, their perceptions of themselves as a person, etc.

So the person Psycho-Social structures are in disarray at this time.

The person now needs to cope with this and at the same time develop new Psycho-Social structures that can cope with a life without using alcohol.

> This part is not as neat and simple as the clinical detox. And this is the part that makes a difference between Success and Failure.

To see what has happened here look at the following.

We began where it was normal for the body to have zero alcohol. This was the Normal State.

Then we introduced alcohol to the body and the Pattern of Consumption and the Psycho-Social learning process began.

Once alcohol was being consumed, the usage increased and the person began to use it regularly.

Regular use became the new Normal State.

Then we increased the consumption level and frequency to 1.5 bottles of wine daily. Then this became the new Normal State.

Then; when we Ceased Consumption of the alcohol, the body protested because we changed what it was by then conditioned to do.

That new conditioning was to process, manage and handle alcohol at the level of 100 units of alcohol a week or 1.5 bottle of wine a day.

Then we said that we would halt that drinking behaviour!

Instead of going through a process of gradually reducing the amount of alcohol, we immediately removed it.

And the body did not have any opportunity to adjust to the removal of the alcohol.

This is Clinical Substance Addition where the body is physically in need of alcohol to maintain its Normal State.

Physical Clinical Addition is actually a fairly easy process to understand and deal with.

For example;

Physical Clinical Addiction to alcohol can be dealt with in 7 days.

Within 7-days the body goes through the withdrawal from alcohol dependency and is no longer clinically dependent upon alcohol.

Medication may be used during the withdrawal period to make the withdrawal process easier and to prevent the potentially dangerous fits which can occur.

However this does not mean that the person's problems that they have with; and which are associated with alcohol, have ceased.

We may have dealt with the Physical Addiction component but there is still the Psycho-Social component to deal with; and this is usually more complicated and messy.

The Habits and Behaviours Associated With the Addictive Behaviour.

A failure to deal with the Psycho-Social components adequately, usually leads the person back to their previous behaviour or to behaviour of a similar type and degree.

It can be around the time at which the clinical addiction is being dealt with that other problems can occur; such as switching addiction from one substance to another, or to another type of behaviour.

Switching addiction is problematic because someone may appear to have dealt with the problem but what is happening is that they are seeking another quick way of managing things.

At a surface level it can appear that the person is dealing with the problems well and they can appear to be making remarkable progress using the new coping structures.

Whereas in reality; they are likely to have just found something else to focus on for a while, and this can act to absorb stress; for a while.

> I have seen this a number of times and seen people crash and return to previous behaviours with a vengeance.
>
> As a therapist you have to watch out for this and deal with it with the person; if you can.

Post Addiction.

This later part; Post Addiction (afterwards), should be familiar to many dieters! I have written it to include food.

> The Psycho-Social behaviour is usually the part of the problem that takes time and can be very complicated and difficult to deal with.
>
> The Psycho-Social component has to be dealt with in the real world of the person and in real time.
>
> In their real world they would have had Psycho-Social exposure to Foods over a period of time. Often many years and decades.
>
> As part of this process they would have been exposed to different behaviours around Food as they grew up and socialised with other people and different foods.
>
> Some of that exposure to different behaviours would be Positive and some would have been Negative. And some of it would have been Messed-up and Corrupted.
>
> Throughout this process they would be learning and copying.
>
> Where they have no clear directions they will have made up their own behaviours and established their own internal mechanisms for managing Life issues.

A note about Addictive Substances.

> Now it doesn't matter what liquid or solid is consumed by the person; it is the active Alcohol content of what they consume that is taken in and processed by the body.
>
> So wine, beer, spirits, alcohol based mouth wash, alcohol based perfumes, puddings with alcohol in, etc; all have the base component (ingredient) of Alcohol in them which will be picked up and processed by the body.
>
> The bodies processing of alcohol, even in very small quantities, can trigger links which will take the person back to and beyond previous levels of consumption with alcohol.
>
> It can also trigger links to previous behaviours related to the Psycho-Social components. This can then lead to behavioural changes which have a tendency to take the person back to their previous behaviour.
>
> This is also true about drugs and other addictive substances.

So although someone may deal with their clinical addiction, something within them has changed as a result of becoming addicted.

In my view; that change remains in place like a Sensitivity which can easily be disturbed.

Hidden Substances

Now there is another component to this section which is:

> Substances that we may consume without knowing that we are consuming them.
>
> And having consumed them over time; we have become used to having them in our bodies.
>
> If we then change the food that we eat, we may experience a reaction to the fact that this substance has been removed.

This type of reaction has occurred over the years with things like Tranquillisers.

People took the Tranquilisers under medical supervision only to find that they had extreme physical, and sometimes psychological, reactions when they changed medication or stopped taking the medication.

Over time it was discovered that components within the medication had addictive qualities that were not appreciated at the time.

Is it possible that this could occur with foods?

In reality almost anything is possible. That however does not make it probable.

Let's look at what I think is more likely.

Consuming More – The New Normal!

Now we know that foods have components such as sugars.

In normal quantities sugars do not present problems for most people.

In larger quantities sugars create a problem for most people.

For the normal functioning of the body we consume sugars in different forms along with fats and other materials.

We know that we can Over Provide our bodies with substances (such as Food) which then causes our bodies to process them; and manage the consequences of consuming them.

If we Over Provide on a regular basis then our bodies will also go through an adjustment where it needs to handle Above Normal Amounts.

Keep this up for a long enough period of time and you adjust the Normal State of the body from one of handling Normal Amounts of food (Green Zone); to one of having to handle Larger than Normal amounts of food or consumed items (Amber or Red Zones).

So for the person who Over Provides their body with food; the New Normal becomes one of Consuming More!

And as a result of Consuming More:

> They move out of the Green Zone and into the Amber and Red Zones for Food Consumption.

Once you have change the bodies Normal State to one of Consuming More, and you then take away the increased consumption; such as what happens when someone goes on a diet, certain things are bound to happen.

> When you remove the Increased Consumption; your body then has to go through an adjustment period while it adjust to the severe reduction in food.

Now this Adjustment Period may take some time to work through and it could be months.

> During this period you may well feel very uncomfortable, as if you are missing something fundamental from your life.
>
> You may feel as if your life is in turmoil.
>
> You may well feel hungry all the time and even completely ravenous.

Of course you would; because you have ceased to do what has become Normal behaviour for you and you have done something “Not Normal” for you.

> You have moved out of the Over Supply Range; which is normal for you. And you have moved into the Under Supply Range which is not normal for you.

Now we know that Change is normally a stressful process that can be unpleasant.

At the time of dieting you are changing something fundamental to Your Lifestyle in a drastic way by going on a diet.

For most people a diet involves doing something completely different, and often demanding, which involves different foods and behaviours.

In reality; when people diet, they are attempting to do two physically demanding things at the same time: Which are actually somewhat Contradictory.

They want to:

> Change their eating habits and change their practices with food.
>
> And at the same time:
>
> Reduce their food intake. Stop putting on weight and begin Losing weight.
>
> So: *Change their Normal State by rapidly reversing and changing their normal practices with food.*

For most people on a diet these Must Occur at the same time and Must both produce positive results.

Putting these two things together simply compounds the difficulty of the process and reduces the probability of success.

If you then throw exercise into the mix; and that they are attempting to change embedded behaviours that have developed over time. Their stress is now going to be very high.

Then if we ask the question:

> How have they previously responded to stressful situations?

Usually they will have been using the consumption of food and other behaviours related to food to do this.

> Which they have now drastically tried to changed or remove from their life.

So the stage is now set for failure and they are probably not long into the new diet.

We are also now in a position where we can see another Human Dynamics playing itself out:

The Yo-Yo Dieting Process.

So is this Food Addiction or is it something else?

Personally I do not think it is Food Addiction as I currently understand it.

This is similar to Addiction to a Substance but is not the same as it.

There is no single substance or single group of substances that the person is consuming on a regular enough basis, or in quantities which have the profile to form an addiction.

> Being hungry and requiring nourishment, sustenance and nutrition might make us ravenous; but this is easily satisfied by many different types of food.
>
> Satisfying hunger in this way is not the same as satisfying the addiction when alcohol is removed.

In this process I think we are dealing with Psycho-Social components which have become interwoven with food consumption and the habits and structures around food.

I think that it is a Problem Mix where food and food related behaviour has become Over-Used in different ways; and that has created problems.

One of those problems is that the body has adjusted it's Normal State from being one of dealing with less food; to a Normal State of dealing with Consuming More; or an Over Supply of food.

If we compare the process that I used earlier with Addiction to alcohol, and compare this to the Consuming More State; it will be similar but different in a significant way.

A Food related example would look like this: It may begin with, for example, that someone is not very confident, is shy, nervous, feels like they don't fit in, are unhappy, etc.

They find that eating and the behaviour around food and eating, helps them to feel better and to have some form of control when faced with certain situations, feelings or emotions.

This process can lead to the release of hormones within the body that produce the "feeling better" affect.

The person then has an altering relationship with Food which, over time, leads on to changes with their Use and Consumption of Foods.

> And over time this behaviour becomes over used and then problematic through the consequences that it produces.

As this Food related process is developing and becoming problematic; other things in their lives are changing as well, such as their physical appearance.

So in my view it becomes Dependency and a Psycho-Social problem rather than Addiction.

Let's put this into the context of the Green, Amber and Red Zones from the Dieters Scale© that we looked at earlier.

Someone would begin their relationship with food in the Green Zone, then progress towards the Amber Zone as their normal food consumption changed;

and then they would move into the Red Zone as their normal food consumption changed once more.

Not only would they move through the different Zones for food consumption, they would also move through the different Zones for Relationships, Work, Confidence, Self-Esteem, etc.

As a consequence the overall Pattern of someone's Life alters gradually over time!

And this is what ends up needing to be changed:

The Pattern of someone's Life!

Note
We can become addicted or biased towards the release of certain hormones in the body and an example of this can be from behaviour that tends to become extreme.

Examples of this are behaviour like Base Jumping, very high levels of Sex, Gambling, Dangerous Activity with very high risk factors, etc.

People who do these activities say: They love the High or Rush that they achieve.

Once again these activities can begin innocently but then become corrupted as a means of achieving and providing more than they are able to give.

Consuming Less and Less

In the previous example I have used Increased Food Consumption which focuses on people who are overweight.

For those who are Underweight, I think that the same processes apply but we are working with the other end of the Spectrum of Weight Problems.

Eating less becomes their New Normal.

Their Normal State is changed from eating in the Normal Range (Green Zone) to eating Outside of the Normal Range (In the Amber and Red Zone).

Eventually someone will move from the Green Zone and take up Residence in the Amber Zone; and then in the Red Zone.

As they progress through the zones the scale, complexity and difficulty of their problem mix is likely to increase.

When it comes to the time to change eating behaviours from Consuming Less to Consuming More; the same uncomfortable processes occur.

Most people will take years to develop their problem mix to a point where they are Properly Motivated to finally do something Positive about it.

So it stands to reason that to be able to successfully address such problems so as to Improve, Resolve or Better Manage them; that it will also take time and effort.

Changing how we Feel!

Whether we are looking at substances which are introduced into the body, like alcohol, drugs and food.

Or; whether we are talking about substances that the body produces as a result of behaviour, such as; having a really good time, Sex, or extreme sports.

What we are really concerned with is:

Changing how we feel through an activity or experience.

If we are looking to change how we feel then we are looking at:

Altering moods.
Altering emotions.
Altering feelings.
Altering behaviour.
Altering consequences.

All of these can lead on to:

Substance addiction.
Behavioural Dependency.
Substance dependency.

It is my view that everyone can live a better and more positive life:

> If they want to and are prepared to do what is required to do so.

I think that many people with persistent weight problems are actually making a very strong request for help when they go on a diet.

Unfortunately they often try to put too many conditions on the help that they want.

I invite you, as someone who diets, to make this the beginning of a new style of Living and Being.

A new start where you can deal with the realities of Life without turning to food to provide the help, comfort and support that you need.

Instead you will use the new tools and structures that are available for you, to help you have a better quality and more successful life in the future.

Go on; Go for it!

If we accept the fact that we want to improve our lives, feel better about our lives and how we live them; then we can address this in a more Positive Way.

It is often when we are being Passive that we develop Negative Habits; rather than Positive Habits.

To be a successful person we need to be Pro-Active.

Anyone, at any age, regardless of any life factors can be Pro-Active.

So what do I want you to take away from this chapter?

In the development and maintenance of a weight problem there are many different components.

We can look for exotic justifications for our problems but the reality is that the causes of our problems are usually more mundane and simple:

> We are not using food and the consumption of food in the right way, for the right reasons, at the right times.

As well as the behaviour related to food, there is a basket of other issues which also develops.

These other issues can become more complicated and difficult to understand than the weight problem.

The longer that all this goes on, the more difficult it becomes to deal with it all.

Eventually people lose sight of the things that have happened in the past and just begin to focus on the Consequences that they are experiencing today.

As a result they then become focused on dealing with the consequences of the problem and not the causes.

As a result the consequences can continue for many years.

When you deal with the causes; you disempower the consequences.

CHAPTER 7

Permanently Changing Your Life Profile For Food, Etc.

I am including this chapter because I want people to understand something about how we create and influence our own lives.

We do this through our previous Life Experiences and how we have Internalised and Used those experiences.

If we have created Faulty Internalised material then we need to be able to change it.

There is a process which is involved in this; and that we all use; but which we don't all know about.

I hope that this explanation will help you to understand about the Internalisation Process and how it actually affects you.

I am going to use the device of a book and the structure of a book to do this.

So think of your Life Experiences being put into a book and creating chapters and pages in a book called:

Your Life Profile.

So what is "Your Life Profile"?

An easy way to think of it is like this.

Imagine that when you are born you are given a book. And this book is going to tell your Life Story but in a different way to normal.

Instead of looking in at your life from the outside world perspective. This book is about how you experience and interact with the world from the Inside Out.

So this book contains your Inner World Experiences and Perspective of things.

> This book contains the experiences, knowledge, insights and other important things which together create the structure of your life and which shape you as a person.

As you go through your life, you will experience new things which can affect you and which help to create the person you are.

As a result of those experiences new chapters are created in your book and new pages are added to those chapters.

For example:

> Going to school creates a new chapter.
>
> Adolescence creates another. Our bodies are developing, we become self-conscious and we are vulnerable to comments and observations made by others.

Each of these significant episodes creates their own chapter which help to inform how comfortable we are with things like showing our bodies to others.

Then there are the chapters on Relationships which we develop as we become older.

And the chapters on our various life experiences; the holidays we have enjoyed, the places we have lived, the people we have met.

Then there are the chapters on Loss. The people and things which we lose as part of the process of living.

Now if we experienced difficulties in life with things like Bullying then different things can happen.

Certain parts of the Life Experiences we have had may become a part of our distant past but other parts can still connect with us today.

These experiences remain present in our lives and become a part of our Life Structure.

Your Dieting and the different Positive and Negative experiences you have had with dieting and food also create their own chapters and pages.

As you use and misuse a new substance or behaviour it creates a new chapter or adds new pages in the index of the book called:

Your Life Profile.

As a result those chapters which are being used all the time, take up more space and have more information for you to refer back to and act upon.

Eventually you will have lots of different chapters that tell the story of your Life history and the different behaviours and different activities associated with it.

Now the place where all these different chapters of Your Life Profile are stored is in your Mind, your Body, your Spirit and in your Lifestyle.

> They now help to shape and control who and what you are!

Many of the chapters in Your Life Profile will merge together and form the foundation for who and what you are as a person.

However; not all the chapters will merge together.

Certain Chapters in Your Life Profile are going to be different from the others.

We will call these the Special Chapters.

The Special Chapters

The Special Chapters are different because they have caused or can cause something to change at a Fundamental Level in your life.

These changes can be both Positive and Negative in the results they produce.

What I want to focus on at this point is the one that troubles us: The Negative.

> Now what you need to understand here is that although this is Your Life Profile; you are not always in charge of this thing.
>
> It will operate on its own and with or without your Cognitive Support (Your awareness of giving support to thoughts or actions that you take).

In fact Your Life Profile develops chapters which tells it how to operate and what to do when you are Confused, Uncertain, Unhappy, Undecided, Nervous, etc.

Think of these chapters as being like a Hand-Book or Instruction Manual.

Whether you make a Conscious Decision to do something or not; Your Life Profile will check out the Special Chapters to see what to do and how to do it.

The more Your Life Profile refers to those Special Chapters, the more influence and control that they have and the more you will follow them without question.

> And Yes! This includes the chapters that you have for Diets and Food.

Now what you have to realise is that once a chapter has been created; it can't be removed. It is there, it exist, it has happened.

So for a dieter; you cannot remove your dieting history and the behaviours associated with it.

For someone who has become Addicted to Drugs and Alcohol; their Chapters on these substances cannot be removed and will always exist.

I think that this is one of the most important things for you to understand:

> Once something is in Your Life Profile it cannot be removed.
>
> However; you can write New Chapters.
>
> And you can write New Special Chapters!
>
> And you can change how you use the existing chapters.

And that is what this book is all about.

It's about Writing New Special Chapters in Your Life Profile so that we can use them to change your future.

And this is where many people make mistakes!

Instead of writing New Special Chapters, what they actually do is they write more pages for the existing ones; usually the Negative ones.

This just makes the existing ones bigger and more influential; and this then causes them to repeat the same behaviour and achieve the same results.

So going from one diet plan to another diet plan will add new pages and new chapters to the Weight Control and Diet Plan Index in Your Life Profile.

The result is that you make the Weight Problem section bigger!

My question to you is:

Are you ready to write New Special Chapters for Your Life Profile that influences and affects your weight problem in a Positive and Beneficial way?

Or:

Do you want to continue to re-enforce all the things which do not work, which harm you long term and which make you Unhappy?

So what do I want you to take away from this chapter?

Your dieting history and your associated problems are written into Your Life Profile.

At the start of each day, you have a choice to continue to write more pages into the existing chapters of Your Life Profile or not.

To deal with a long term weight problem and the associated issues; you need to write new Special Chapters and positive pages in Your Life Profile.

We can all do this with the right help and support.

CHAPTER 8

Stop Measuring The Symptom: Your Weight. And Start Measuring Other Things.

When I have worked with people who have problems that involve their weight. I have found that many of them have become conditioned to weighing themselves and measuring themselves.

The frequency with which they do this does not take account of normal physical variability and the effects of this upon measured weight.

Measuring too often and in the wrong way is a Counter-Productive Process which produces ongoing Negative Re-enforcement.

My view is:

> Let your weight be an indicator that you can use in a positive way, rather than a stick with which to beat yourself.

Nature has given us methods by which we can tell if we are growing in the wrong direction.

However; the marketing and sales of diet products and diet solutions, needs us to focus on a benchmark that they can successfully use to get us to buy their products.

And a quick and easy benchmark is your weight and your size.

And you are going to be sensitive to one or the other or both of these, when you have a problem with your weight and the other issues that go along with it.

Now I am not saying that the Diet Industry is to blame for your weight problem or for how you measure your weight.

However; your Psycho-Social Education will have been exposed to lots of input from these areas and they will have influenced you; whether you realise it or not.

Just think of how many newspapers and magazines you have looked at where Looks and Appearance mattered?

How many television programmes, news reports and films have you seen where Looks and Appearance mattered?

How many conversations have you listened to or taken part in where Looks and Appearance matters?

All of this adds to your Psycho-Social Education and it can make you more and more Sensitive to these issues.

> Do you think that it is a coincidence that the Diet Industry offers people a fast and easy way to lose weight quickly?

The reality is that people want this and so they are offered it.

What most people don't realise is that this is, in effect; A Trick!

It is quite easy to lose those first few pounds over a few weeks.

Put a simple process in place to achieve this and you can call it a diet plan.

By the time someone starts on a new diet they are often so fed up with how they have been that they are desperate for something different.

Give them a little bit of weight loss or the loss of inches from certain parts of their bodies and they are happy.

However: Being able to maintain that weight loss and those good feelings into the future is another matter.

> The reality is that the front end of a weight problem is usually the easiest to address – at least in the early stages.

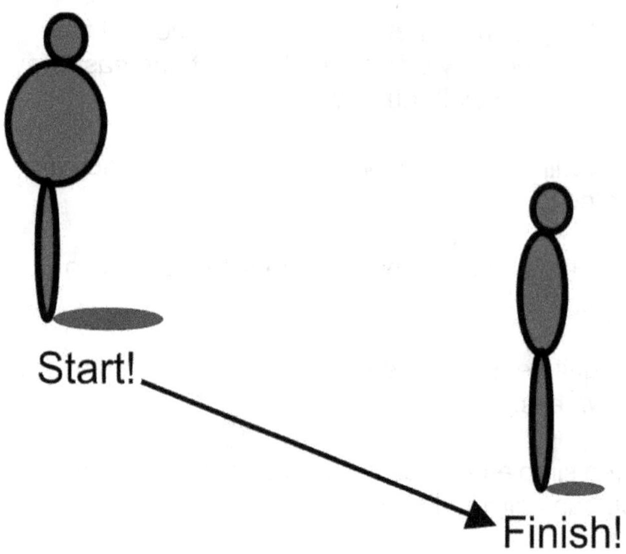

Diet plans are often sold on the basis of losing so much weight a week or a month.

The only problem with this plan is that Your Body didn't get the memo which told it that it should behave in that fashion.

And the reality is that your body doesn't work like that.

Weight loss and weight gain is not a simple linear process as illustrated in the picture above.

It tends to be a process which involves Positive and Negative moves with your weight over time.

I think that a better way to view the long term dieting process is illustrated in the next graphic.

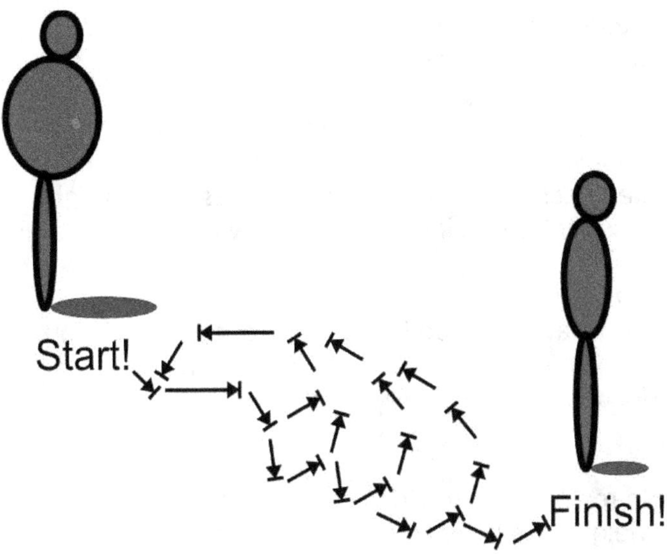

Let's see if any of this is familiar to you?

I have seen people:

Use weighing scales; measure the circumferences' of different parts of their bodies; put themselves into wraps to squeeze themselves into different shapes; and try to squeeze themselves into different sized clothing (often with the help of sturdy undergarments).

Stories of people not eating before going for a weight-in and then pigging out afterwards are common.

Stories of people going to the toilet and taking laxatives and diuretics before a weight-in are common.

Stories of people taking off their clothes before a weight-in are common.

These are just simple examples of what lengths people will go to, so that they can be told that they have achieved some form of success with weight loss; or look as if they have lost weight.

So what advice do I give to the people that I work with on a Life Improvement Programme that focuses on Weight Problems?

In reality sustainable weight gain and sustainable weight loss is measured over months, years and decades. Not in days and weeks.

A more accurate way to think of weight control is:

> That we acquire and have Tendencies to either Gain weight, Lose weight or Maintain weight.
>
> And we may, according to the influences of other factors, move from one Tendency to another.
>
> And at any one time, we are going to be living in One Tendency as regards our weight.
>
> We will be Living In the Tendency for:
>
> - Increasing weight.
> - Losing weight.
> - Maintaining weight.

If we are Living In the wrong Tendency for what we want to achieve; then we need to move to another one.

Moving into another Tendency takes time!

When I work with someone on a Life Improvement Programme that is focused on Weight.

I help them to move from the Tendency for fast short term results, to the Tendency for sustainable longer term results.

When we do this we have to take account of the fact that the person is going to live for many years (baring illness and accidents).

We want to achieve some short term benefits but our eyes should be on the future – focused on the person living the life that they really want to live!

Working with Tendencies is a longer term game.

As well as working with the persons Tendencies related to their weight; we also work with their Tendencies in other areas of their lives such as their Self-Esteem.

I do this because weight problems do not exist in a vacuum.

I mentioned earlier that:

> Nature has given us methods by which we can tell if we are growing in the wrong direction.

So I like to use these methods and in reality they are simple.

As we begin a Life Improvement Programme, I would want to know personal details such as someone's actual weight.

After that I am not really interested in their actual weight until we reach certain milestones; and then only to have accurate information.

I am more interested in:

- How easy the person finds it to move?
- How their clothes are fitting?
- Do they feel better as they get up and sit down in chairs and use other furniture?
- Are they feeling healthier?
- What are their Emotions doing?
- How are they Feeling about themselves.
- What they are doing that feels different?
- How are they sleeping?
- Are they looking in mirrors?

And other aspects of their behaviours related to food and the consequences of having a problem with their weight.

If we do things like this, we don't have that same pressure that we experience with a regular weigh-in.

I also discourage people from regularly weighing themselves. Even though, in the early days, people still tend to continue to do so.

Other issues that we will address include things like:

- Cyclical weight gain.
- The physical realities of weight gain and weight loss.
- Genetic realities.

I find that this approach takes us in the Right Direction and it takes us to the Right Long Term Outcome.

So what do I want you to take away from this chapter?

Weighing yourself too often means that you are Living In the wrong Long Term Tendency.

To move into the Right Long Term Tendency takes time and you need to write some new chapters in Your Life Profile to help you with this.

Weight problems are as much a Mind problem as a Body problem. As such both of these need to be worked with.

CHAPTER 9

Genetic Realities

"Your mind is writing cheques
that your body can't pay."

When you were born your genetics were provided to you through your parents genetic mix. This mix provided you with your own unique genetic profile.

You have scope within your genetic profile for variations in different areas.

Things like how tall we grow will be influenced by our genetics and access to medical treatment, food and exercise.

Once we have used the genetic tools that we were born with and we have developed and exploited their Potential; it is usually not possible to change things.

For example: If someone with good food, exercise and health grows to 6 feet tall; they cannot reduce their size to 5 feet tall or grow to 7 feet tall.

Their Potential for Physical growth contained within their genetics has been exploited fully and cannot be reversed.

With other things we also have genetic components and we have scope for variation with the Potential of those components.

The Potential is the range within which something can develop and grow. For example:

> Our senses are something that can be honed and developed. We can build muscles, learn to run faster, run further, lift more, etc.

Our Physical Weight is also one of those things where we have scope for variation.

Our weight can vary over a Potentially wide range.

We can survive over this wide weight range and we can even go to extremes of it for long periods.

> However; we will probably experience consequences as a result of exposure to these extremes if they last too long.

Now some people naturally have the genetic ability to be slim and some people naturally have the genetic ability to be large.

A great number of us fit somewhere between the two.

The reality is that if you have the genetic ability to be large and you feed that ability; then you will become large.

Once you have become large and your body has adjusted to Being Larger.

Then this is: The New You.

You have changed the profile of your body.

You may not like the result but this has not happened over night; you would have worked at developing it over time.

> If you don't like what you have created and you want to change it.
>
> What you then have to do is work with the profile of the New You and the Potential for changing this new profile.

It is pointless longing after your past profile because it has now changed. That is the Past You!

The Potential for change that we have includes:

Physical improvements.
Psychological changes.
Behaviour changes.
Emotional improvements.
Perceptual changes.
Environmental changes.

Now let's do something stupid. Let's take an example from the Animal World to explore this.

Let's take a large African elephant.

Most people knows what an elephant looks like.

It's one of those big grey things with tusk, a long trunk and big ears. Oh yeah; it has one of those stupid little tails at the back.

Now imagine that our elephant is being a normal elephant and it becomes as big as its genetics and its access to food and water allows it to become.

Then imagine that one day our elephant comes across a Rhino running through the grass and thinks: Wow!

Our elephant thinks how elegant that Rhino is. How slim and attractive and fit it is.

Our elephant thinks: I want to be just like that Rhino!

Now we all know that the elephant is never going to be just like that Rhino.

They are different species, different body types, different sizes, different capacities, different capabilities.

If the elephant compared itself to another elephant then it may be able to do something; but to a Rhino!

So now let's say that the elephant sets about becoming just like the rhino that it so admired.

The elephant's mind is now writing cheques that its body cannot pay!

People do this same sort of thing in all walks of life, in all forms of activity and in all fields of endeavour.

A great example is when you watch children playing.

They want to be the super hero that flies through the skies.

They want to be the monster that comes from the seas.

They want to be the doctor that operates and saves the day.

They want to be the policeman, spaceman, fireman, etc.

However; no sane adult would actually let the child perform a real operation, try to arrest a real criminal, tackle a real fire or get on a real rocket ship into space.

As adults; we can see the difference between the healthy imaginings of a child and the reality of doing these things.

However; sometimes these things do take a turn for the worse, and sometimes with fatal consequences, when children actually begin to believe that they can fly or that they can jump from tall buildings.

The child's mind begins to write cheques that their body cannot pay. And catastrophic outcomes can follow.

Of course adults and teenagers know better!

- They are not going to have unrealistic expectations; are they?

- They are not going to look at themselves in the mirror and see a fantasy image of themselves; are they?

- They are not going to look at other people as if they are some form of super hero; are they?

Of course they are!

Except they are not looking at children playing in a park; they are looking at themselves through the perspective of their own insecurities, fears, anxieties, tiredness, frustrations, wants, needs and desires.

This process of comparing and wishing to be like someone else, is almost guaranteed to give those with any form of imagination a platform for Self-Deception and Self-Deprecation.

A platform where we see ourselves, life and ourselves within life; in some distorted shapes, sizes and perceptions.

And it is this that takes us to the point where:

Our minds are writing cheques
that our bodies can't pay!

We lose the ability to see the Comparative Realities of what we really can achieve; and we begin to lust after those which we cannot.

And so many people don't realise that this Human Dynamic exist or that they have, in fact, become caught in the fantasy world that they thought they had left behind as children.

Except this is not a children's world; it is the world of Being Human.

And this is a world that we can negotiate and navigate through in successful ways.

> I developed the Human Dynamics Matrix to help me negotiate and navigate through this.
>
> To help us see that which is not so obvious but which has real world consequences for us.

Let's see if we can stop our minds writing cheques that our bodies cannot cash.

Let's focus on writing cheques that we can cash!

So what do I want you to take away from this chapter?

Have the wisdom to know the difference between what you can really change and what you can't change.

Have the courage to change what you can and to live with what cannot be changed.

Focus on where you want to go with your life and not where you have been.

Stop allowing your mind to write cheques that your body cannot cash!

CHAPTER 10

Finding Your Seed Of Belief!

I figure that if you are reading this book; then you are looking for something that you haven't found yet.

I am hoping that either through this book, my other books or through one of my Life Improvement Programmes; that I can help you to find and achieve what you want.

A lot of what I am looking at and exploring in this book, relates to the structure of Persistent Weight Problems and the structure of the Solution that the Persistent Weight Problems require to be successfully resolved, improved or better managed.

The reason for this is that I want this book to do something different for you, than all the other Weight Control, Diet books and Programmes that you have tried in the past.

I am going to let you into a secret.

I am trying to touch a part of your mind
that knows the reality of the situation; and that
wants to work with that reality.

Let me give you some background to what it is that I am trying to do when I work with people.

In the early 1990's: When I worked with people who had long term weight problems, I found that all the people that I saw had problems with sleeping.

They either found it difficult to get to sleep, have a good quality of sleep or both.

At the time I had trained and practiced as a Hypnotherapist.

However; I did not agree with how people were marketing Hypnotherapy and the claims that they were making for it. *(I still don't today)*

Personally; I just seemed to view Hypnotherapy, and the potential benefits that it could provide, in a different way to my Peers. And I just could not make claims that I did not support or believe in.

So I went my own way with the Principles of Hypnotherapy.

I knew that Hypnotherapy could be used in beneficial ways but I just did not believe in the quick fix claims.

Too many of the problems that people were claiming could be cured, improved or resolved by the use of Hypnotherapy were not sustainable.

People could feel better through its use; but to claim that you were able to change, often quite substantial things, by simple suggestion through one or two Hypnotherapy sessions: I just did not see the evidence for that.

My view has always been, and still is, that if an Alternate Therapy approach is as good as people claim it is; then it will have Predictability of Outcome.

And when I work with Weight related problems and other types of problems, this is what I am interested in:

> Predictability of Outcome. And;
>
> The Processes for successfully achieving it.

Predictability of Outcome means that you should be able to say:

- That if I have a person with (X) condition/situation.
- And I apply (Y solution) in this way.
- Over this period of time.
- Then I would expect to achieve (Z) Outcome.
- To a degree (%) of success.
- If the person does their bit along the way.

So let's get back to my secret.

When it comes to problems I have always been interested in the Predictability of the Outcome.

I knew that I was working with people who had a long dieting history.

These were people from different backgrounds, who had lived in different countries and who had a wide range of ages.

Some had been successful or were currently successful in their careers and others had normal occupations and incomes.

Most of them were women.

I knew that they had tried many diets and programmes and many had achieved successful results from them.

But!

Despite being successful with various diet plans, weight control programmes and programmes that provided calorie controlled meals.

None of these people had been able to maintain and then build upon the success that they had achieved with their dieting and weight control programmes.

They had all gone back to their previous weights and some had gone a long way past.

What these people really wanted to achieve but didn't actually realise it was:

They wanted to Be Truly Successful In Life!

Being the right weight and being unhappy is not the successful result that people want. It's not substantial enough.

Being successful with your weight but not being successful with your Life; is not really the type of success that most people want.

They want both of these things together! They want:

> To be in control of their weight and to be successful with managing it.
>
> And
>
> To Be truly successful in their lives.

Being truly successful in your life means living the life that you want and that you are happy living. Or that you are moving in the right direction to achieve this.

So let's get back to my secret.

At that time, in the 1990's, I had spend several years working with Alcohol and Drug problems with a Charity and also with a multi-disciplinary medical team that ran a Community Alcohol Programme (CAT). I had trained as a Counsellor.

I could see from my own experiences that there were Commonalities between Alcohol, Drugs and Weight problems and many other conditions.

Over a period of time I was able to identify common issues across the range of different problems.

These common issues included: Self-Esteem, Confidence, Self-Perceptions, Motivation, etc.

I call these common issues:

The Basket of Common Components.

This is because they tend to be Common Components of the structure that makes up difficult and complex problems.

As a result of this work, I then knew that if someone came to me with a long term weight problem, that I could expect them to have the basket of common components and also their own specific issues.

So I had all these people who had problems with sleeping. And I had this tool called Hypnotherapy.

To me, Hypnotherapy was a tool that could be used better in the mid to long term, in a progressive way; rather than in the short term or very short term.

So I began developing a way to use it this way.

Because of the availability of audio equipment I decided that I would write, record and mix an audio programme for the people with weight problems.

So I created and produced a 6 cassette programme that I had designed to be used over a 3 month period.

It probably took me about 6 months to do this.

My plan was that I would use this audio programme to help establish a better sleeping pattern for the people I was working with.

I also wanted to use the audio programme to help them with relaxation and give them something different to focus on.

What I also wanted to do was to begin working with the common basket of problems through the audio programme and the one-to-one sessions we were having.

And this is my secret!

There was something that I observed and picked up on when I was working with and interviewing people with persistent weight problems.

That thing was:

> That they Hoped that the New Diet approach would work;
>
> But they actually didn't really Believe that it would.

As a result of their previous experiences and their inability to maintain results long term:

They had lost their Seed of Belief.

So I began a process of helping them to Discover their Seed of Belief. The Belief that this time:

It could work!
It could be different!

I did not tell them that we were doing this and I had very good reasons for not doing so. I won't go into those here.

I found that the audio programme helped change people's sleeping habits. Once people sleep better they also feel better. This then helps to facilitate the work that we then need to do.

The result I experienced was that those who persisted with the programme went on to change their relationships with their weight, food, and to change and improve other aspects of their lives.

It is very rewarding as a Therapist to have a client succeed and become independent of you.

Achieving this was not an easy process. There was lots of hard work with little reward over many years.

At that time I was still to invent, innovate, create and develop the material which I am now making available through my books and programmes.

What I was doing, without realising it, was that I was laying the foundations for the work that I would do in the future with The Human Algorithm® Project.

So what do I want you to take away from this chapter?

There is a difference between Wanting something and Knowing that you can obtain it.

I want people with persistent weight problems to Know that they can obtain the result that they want; but these results are part of a Package.

You can't obtain the result without that Package.

The Package that Successful Weight Control and Freedom From Dieting is a part of is:

Being Truly Successful In Life!

It is Moving towards Living the Life that you really want to live; how you really want to live it.

You don't achieve that from a Diet on its own.

CHAPTER 11

Chaos, Chaotic Behaviour And Chaotic Situations.

When I look at different types of problems and when I work with problems, it is not unusual for there to be what I call:

A Chaotic Element.

There are a number of reasons for Chaos, Chaotic Behaviour and Chaotic Situations.

In every situation, each person will give me their view as to "Why" these things exist.

I then go through a process of looking at the real structure of the problem and having to work my way through all the different personal views as to "Why" these problems can't be addressed.

In reality I usually find that it is the Human Component of the problem that is the most difficult to deal with.

The reasons for this include the following:

> That they have been unable to actually deal with the problem and have developed ways of looking at, understanding and working with the Fall-Out from the problem that allows them to cope with the existence of the problem.

They actually don't understand what is going on and they have tried to develop ways of dealing with it; but they can't keep doing so.

They are unwilling to actually deal with the problem because they don't want to have to deal with the associated issues that come with it.

The problem is just Beyond them.

They don't see it as their problem or their area of responsibility; so why should they care about it.

And when I actually begin a process of looking to understand a problem so as to Improve, Resolve or Better Manage it:

I am then challenging what they have done up to that point and many people are Very Sensitive to that process.

This can lead on to:

- Personal Attacks of various sorts.

- The undermining of the Strategy, Processes and Timetable of the solution.

- Infighting, blaming and even Setting-Up people so that they can Change the Dynamics of the solution being applied(to weaken or destroy it).

You see; even though people want things to improve, change and be better:

They are still going to behave as Imperfect People.

- Because we are all Imperfect People.

When we have Chaos, Chaotic Behaviour and Chaotic Situations around for long enough:

They become NORMAL.

And our own behaviours then begin to adjust; and our lifestyles begin to support what has become the New Normal for us.

If we referred back to the chapter where we looked at the Dieters Scale and the Green, Amber and Red Zones. And if we relate that to this subject.

We find that:

> People in Chaos, when they participate in the Chaos, do not Live in the Green Zone.
>
> What they are doing is Living in the Amber or Red Zone.
>
> The Amber and Red Zones have more difficulties associated with them, and more Stress, and they are More Demanding.

So Chaos, Chaotic Situations and Chaotic Behaviour can all be graded into Zones. This process then helps us to understand what we are dealing with.

In my experience there are very few, what I would term, "Real Chaotic" situations; where we cannot achieve Control, Stability and Better Management of the situation.

What I do find is that as people gradually lose control of and over situations; that Chaos moves in and can then become a justification for the persons inability to better manage the situation.

So the chaos is a result of other things and not the cause of other things.

What I have also found to be true is:

> If Chaos is a constant part of the problem; then Chaos becomes predictable.
>
> Once Chaos is predictable it then becomes understandable.
>
> Once it becomes understandable; it then becomes manageable and able to be improved or resolved.

So if we have someone with a persistent weight problem who claims that they cannot do something because things are constantly changing; or that they never know what is going to happen from one day to another; then the reality is that they are living in the Amber or Red Zones.

Because we are Imperfect People we can get ourselves into the situation where:

> Through our own behaviours we find ourselves in situations which are Chaotic.
>
> We then blame the Chaotic situations for our behaviours and for How we are living our lives.
>
> Therefore; the Chaotic situations continue and so do the Negative Consequences.
>
> Over time the degree of difficulty in the situation is also likely to increase; and more areas of the person's life will move into the chaotic Amber and Red Zones.

Once someone becomes Established in the Amber and Red Zones it becomes their Normal; and when we want to change this; we will get all the problems and difficulties that go with changing someone's Normal Behaviour.

From my perspective.

> I have never seen a situation which could not be changed; if the people involved are willing to do what it really takes to improve, resolve or better manage the situation.

Don't be afraid of Chaos. See it for what it is and deal with it as the problem requires you to do so.

So what do I want you to take away from this chapter?

Chaos, Chaotic Situations and Chaotic Behaviours are:

> Problems that have a set of conditions, which are looking for a better way of being managed, so as to produce a more successful result.
>
> David John Sheridan

CHAPTER 12

You Can't Walk Far When You Are Deep In A Hole

The enthusiasm has been building for a while.

Mentally you have been preparing yourself to go on another diet.

In preparation you have put on another few pounds as you eat those things which you know you are going to miss; and that you are not going to be able to eat whilst on the diet.

You even begin limbering up and starting to do a few simple stretching exercises in preparation for getting fit.

Eventually “The Day” arrives and your off!

It's like change-over day at a holiday camp.

Your places in the kitchen become off limits.

Food items may have been moved and hidden; by you.

The off limits food is replaced by the Good Stuff.

All the healthy stuff is there for you to eat and lose weight.

Your daily schedule changes.

In preparation for the weight loss you may even have been out and bought or ordered new clothes; in “The New Size” that you are going to be.

You may have called it “An Incentive”; something to help you focus and get through the difficult times that you know you are going to face.

This may even be an emotional experience for some; like meeting a good friend who has been away for a while and that you are glad to see.

You may even have enlisted the support of others; like you. Friends who have the same wants, needs and desires.

Fellow travellers of the Diet Road.

For those who are in the Green Zone it is more of an even battle.

Those few extra pounds (kilo’s) of weight soon give way to the diet plan and the exercise.

The reward of being slimmer, and feeling fitter and healthier is fantastic. Wow what a buzz!

So how long will the person in the Green Zone keep this up?

Unless they actually like exercise, like I do, then they will reach A Point Of Balance.

A point at which they will weigh up the benefits of being slimmer, and feeling fitter and healthier. And they will weigh this up against the visits to the gym, the disruption to their social life, the inconvenience and costs of their new diet, and the effort to keep this up.

They may also have noticed that the exercise is making them put on weight as they develop muscles.

So this will be the Point of Balance for them.

The Point where they weigh things up and begin to let things slide back to where they were before; or they keep the new habits going.

If we look at those in the Amber Zone.

Well these are more experienced with the dieting process than those in the Green Zone.

They know what to expect and they also will go through their Preparations.

The Amber Zone people will have more "On The Line".

Their physical health issues may have been a motivator for the new diet. Or it may have been Doctors Orders.

This may be "The Opportunity" to sort out your life and the different issues that are Uncomfortably there.

So you begin.

How soon the first crisis or mini-crisis hits depends upon the support structure that the person has managed to put in place.

Do they get over the first crisis or do they want to change the rules of the game; just this once and cheat?

As they move forwards; when do they hit the second mini-crisis, then the third?

Will they hit a forth?

They will also come to a stage where they hit "A Point Of Balance".

The point where they weigh up whether it is worth it.

And then we can ask about those in the Red Zone.

Have they been pushed into another diet?

Is it that they simply must do it and that the consequences of failure are so great that they simply can't be considered?

Is it the last chance for (X)?

And increasingly nowadays:

> Is it time for surgery? As I just can't stop myself and with the help of surgery I am sure that I could. I just need that extra something which makes a difference!

So how can we understand what is actually going on here?

I like to use a simple way of understanding this problem.

The simple way I use is:

You can't walk far
when you are deep in a hole!

Let's apply this to the Green, Amber and Red Zones.

When we begin our lives there is no weight problem, but the tools that we need to develop one are there for us to use.

As we develop within the Green Zone we begin to pick up tools.

And we begin to use those tools.

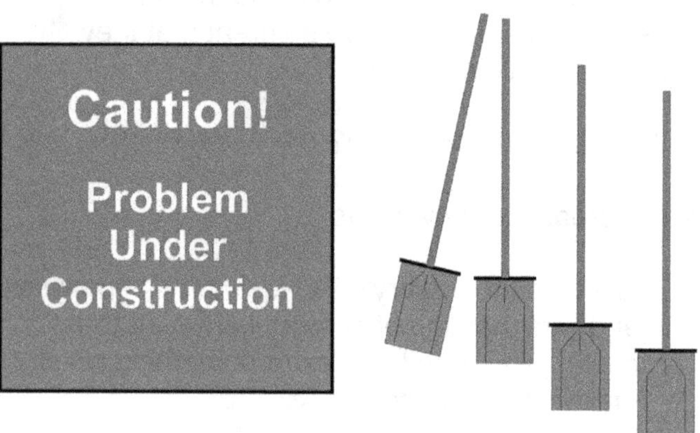

Over time we begin to develop a weight problem and we begin to dig a hole for ourselves.

The tools we use include; Self-Esteem, Confidence, Relationships, Fear, Lack of Direction, etc.

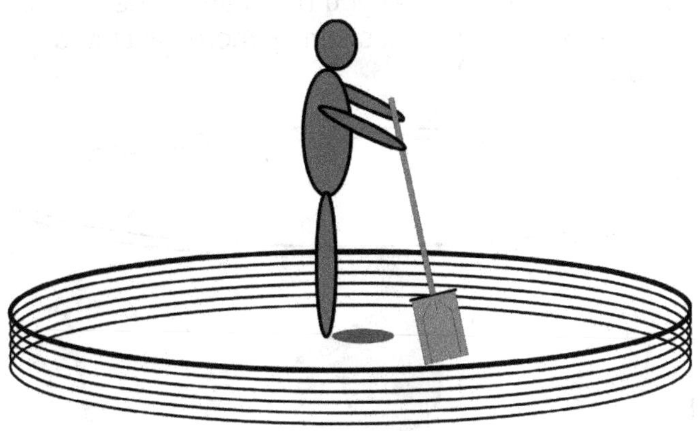

Those who remain in the Green Zone don't dig the hole too deep.

So when they want to deal with all of their weight related problems, it is easier for them to move out of the hole that they have created.

They might trip but they can get out of the hole reasonably easy.

If they fail to move out of the hole then they will stay in it.

If life continues in the same way, then they are in the right place to progress to the Amber Zone.

If we now consider the Amber and Red Zones.

People in the Amber and Red Zones will have gone through the Green Zone and so they are now deeper in the hole.

As a result the hole that you now have to get out of is bigger and deeper. It's simply more difficult to get out of it!

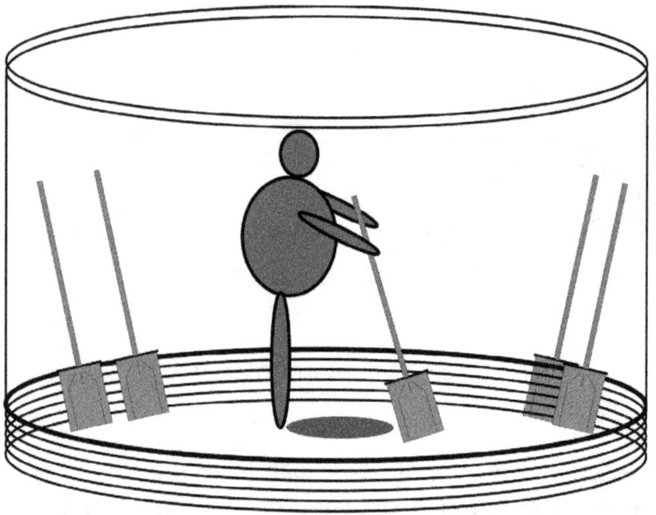

You can see that as the hole gets bigger, that more tools are in the hole.

Each tool represents another issue that relates to the weight problem. These will be either direct or indirectly related issues.

Once you are in the hole, If you put down one tool you can easily pick up another one. So throwing away one tool doesn't work because there are plenty of other tools to hand, and you can't throw them far when you are in a hole anyway.

So thinking that you can get out of the hole by throwing away one diet tool and grabbing another diet tool just gives you another way of staying where you are.

Once you are in deep enough, then you are really:

"In The Hole".

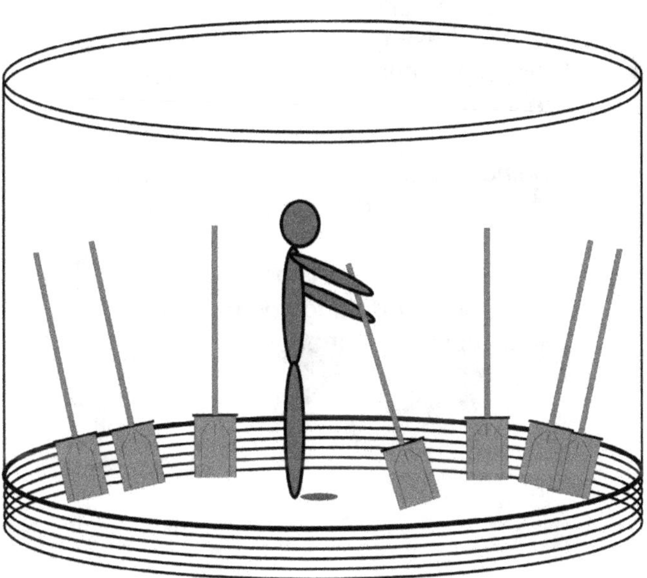

And when you try to get out of the hole, you soon bump into the sides. You can no longer walk out of the hole or easily get out of the hole.

In effect; the whole you have created now defines your life!

So this is why I say:

You can't walk far
when you are deep in a hole!

As you get deeper into the Red Zone the hole just keeps on getting deeper and it can also get wider.

To get out of the hole they have dug for themselves; People tend to try and use the tools that they have and which they are familiar with.

However; they have got into the habit of using these tools in particular ways; which produces certain results.

So: Grabbing the tool of a new diet while you are deep in the hole produces predictable results.

It may be a new diet but it probably won't be giving you anything new or getting you to do anything new; that is substantial enough to make a long term difference.

So what do I want you to take away from this chapter?

As you move from one Zone to another Zone; the nature and structure of the problem that you have changes.

It will have taken you time to dig the hole and as it got deeper you would have shored it up (you build a framework which stops the hole from collapsing in on top of you).

What you used to shored up the hole are all the different things which support and help to maintain the persistent weight problem.

Very often the best thing to do, is to prepare for what you are going to do; but do this in a different way to how you will have done it in the past.

If you are caught in the problem; it will probably be very difficult for you to do this on your own.

> You need to do a combination of changing your tools and the way that you use the tools that you have.
>
> You also need a different plan to the one that you have been using and which has lead to you being in the hole and staying in the hole.

CHAPTER 13

The Reality Of Failure

There are certain activities where failure is part of the process of success. This includes:

All Sports.
All Business.
All of the Sciences.
All of Literature and the Arts.
All Politics.
All Wars.
Peace.
Medicine.
Relationships.
Religion.
Life.

And yet; Dieting and Weight Control are meant to be Failure Free!

All the evidence seems to suggest that this is an untenable and completely unrealistic position.

Failure Free Dieting and Weight Control is a Myth on the same level as Unicorns and Little Green Men from Mars. *(my apologies to Unicorns and little Green Men from Mars if you are reading this.)*

Having the expectation that you must not or will not fail on a diet, puts you under so much pressure that you cannot really succeed.

So rather than waste our time focusing on something which is unachievable; let's scrap it!

Let's accept that you are going to fail! Then let's get beyond it.

You see Failure, in the Right Context, is actually Good!

It says that you are an Imperfect Person who has a problem with your weight and you are working on it.

What I want to do, is get you looking at and working on failure in the right way.

> I use people's failure as a way to understand what was actually going on for them when it happened.
>
> Then we try to make the failure provide a benefit that we can use in a Positive way.

I use different tools to help myself and the person that I am working with; to understand what motivated or produced that failure.

And then we look to deal with it differently when it happens again.

> What we want to do is create New Chapters in Your Life Profile that you can begin referencing and using.
>
> New chapters that have you dealing with failure in new ways.
>
> And new chapters that have you experiencing a better and more successful life.

I think that a better way to think of Weight Control and Dieting is as indicators for:

Being Successful In Life!

Or

Not Being Successful; Yet!

Being Successful In Life!

> Means that you are living the life that you want, in the way that you want; or you are on your way to doing so by taking the Actions that you need to take.

Not Being Successful: Yet!

> Means that you have begun a process of Becoming Successful In Life. And you are beginning to put the structures in place that you will need to achieve your goals.

Remember:

> Your weight is only part of your Sorrow or your Joy!

And that's the way to go about this. Asking yourself the question:

> Are you working on your Sorrow or are you working on your Joy?

If you begin doing this, then I would say that you are beginning to find the Right Path to achieving a

Successful Life that is free from the pressures and disappointments of dieting and weight control.

So what do I want you to take away from this chapter?

Being Perfect all the time is not something that people are good at.

Basically: You can't achieve it and if you can; you can't sustain it.

So it becomes an impossible task.

I prefer to think and act in this way:

> Excellence when required; good enough when appropriate!
>
> Allow yourself to make mistakes and learn from the mistakes that you make.
>
> Failure is often the difference between what you can achieve and what you have achieved.
>
> By seeking excellence when it is required you can often eliminate failure.
>
> Having the wisdom to know the difference between the times when Excellence is required and when Good Enough is appropriate; is achieved by Experience.
>
> Experience is achieved through Doing, Succeeding and Failing. So failure is part of the process of Succeeding!

WHAT'S COMING NEXT!

In the Chapters that follow I am going to look at the Role of certain Common Components within problems that involve Weight.

These are what I would call Life Problems that are common to all of us.

I am not suggesting that you have these problems but I do think that it is worth exploring them in this way.

These problems exist across the entire Spectrum of Weight Problems.

CHAPTER 14

The Role Of Habits In Your Problem

As people, we could not survive without habits.

Habits get us out of bed in the morning, they get us to work and they help us all get along with life.

In every area of our lives we develop habits:

- Lifestyle.
- Wealth.
- Health.
- Well-Being.

Often, because habits are so ubiquitous, we fail to even recognise them as being habits.

Another way of looking at and understanding habits is to think of them as Learned Behaviours. Which is exactly what they are:

> Learned ways of doing things which become automatic.

In fact; most of the time we just drift along in the stream of life and allow ourselves to be moved around without really thinking about it.

Whereas in reality; much of what moves us in our daily lives, is within our control and our ability to influence. It is:

The Habitual Nature of our Lives.

So how would I define a Habit?

If we consider the world that we occupy as a human being, we see that it has different areas which include:

- Emotions/Feelings.
- Psychology (how we process information).
- Actions/Re-actions (how we respond).
- Dynamics (situations in which we find ourselves).
- Other factors.

In each of these areas we are capable of developing and maintaining habits.

Habits are like Short-Cuts.

Rather than have to keep working out how to process, manage or resolve an issue; we do it a few times and then it becomes automatic.

It becomes automatic because at some level it makes sense at the time.

Once it makes sense and it becomes something that we use as part of our make-up as a person; it becomes part of us.

Once it becomes part of us we often tend not to consciously think about what we are doing, why we are doing it or how we are doing it. We just do it!

In fact; thinking about it becomes a chore!

> As Human Beings; we are built so that we do things which we repeat in an automatic fashion. And so much of our lives are repetitions of actions which we repeat.

Now let's consider Habits as Learned Behaviours and use the Dieter's Scale© to understand them better.

On the Dieter's Scale we have Green, Amber and Red Zones.

As we move from the Green Zone to Amber and then to Red, the nature of the problem changes and becomes more complicated and difficult.

Also the Behaviour that occurs within the Amber and Red Zones tends to be less and less Desirable.

So let's use this scale and apply it to habits and Learned Behaviours.

For most people; most of our habits will be in the Green Zone. And many of these will serve us very well and be really useful to us. But not all of them!

As we move into the Amber Zone; these will be habits that can cause us problems and difficulties.

And even though we may be aware of this, we have not changed the habits so as to take them out of the Amber Zone.

In reality: We end up living with them until we have to change them.

As we move into the Red Zone; these will be those habits that cause us most difficulty; one way or another.

Once again we have not changed the habits so as to take them out of the Red Zone.

Now one of the things that we need to understand about habits is this:

> Just because we have developed a habit, it doesn't mean that we know all about it and how to change it.
>
> Often we don't and we can't!

You see; with habits we often lose Perspective!

That old saying: "Can't see the wood for the trees" applies to habits.

You need to remember that the habit has become automatic and that thinking about it becomes a Chore.

So dealing with it, on your own, becomes difficult, and if it is too difficult; we will tend not to deal with it until we really have no choice.

So we put up with it, hoping that it will sort itself out.

This then leads us to the question:

> How can I do something Positive about my Bad habits?

Often we can't see what it is that we are doing and understand why we are doing it.

If we can't see it or understand it; how can we change it?

We need to think of a habit and habitual behaviour as being one and the same thing.

Then it becomes easier to work with.

If we were to sit down and look at the behaviours that you don't like and which you find problematic.

We would find that we can put them into either the Green, Amber or Red Zones.

This would give us a scale for measuring the Problematic Habitual Behaviour and we would expect to handle these differently according to the Zones that they were in.

For example: We would expect that a Green Zone habit would be easier to deal with than an Amber Zone habit.

Now if you decide to take on the hardest and most difficult habit first; then you are taking on the most difficult habitual challenge without any preparation.

So it might be best to tackle something easier to begin with.

Little steps add up to large distances.

In reality; Habits are a necessary part of being human. So you are not going to eliminate habits from your life.

> What we want to do is to change our Tendency from developing and using Bad Habits; to a Tendency for developing and using Good Habits.
>
> So how do we go about doing this?

Remember earlier in this book we had the chapter about Your Life Profile?

Habits are part of Your Life Profile. Habits are what make you use one chapter in Your Life Profile over another.

So what we want to do is to change or modify some habits. And we want to eliminate, reduce or stop using other habits. We also may want to create new habits.

To achieve this we need to be Specific.

- What do we want to change?
- Why do we want to change it?
- What result does this habit produce that we don't want?
- Why are we using this habit in this way?
- How long have we been using this habit?
- Which Zone is this habit in: Red, Amber or Green?

By doing this we can begin to create the Comparative Understanding that we need to change Habitual Behaviour from one thing, to another thing.

Once we begin consciously thinking about these aspects, we can begin to get a proper feeling and understanding of what we are dealing with.

Then we can begin to put "A Plan" together for how we are going to change it.

This Plan would include:

> What steps are we going to take?
> When are we going to do them?
> How do I want to change this habit?
> How long do I think it will take?
> Can I do this on my own or do I need help?

Now something that you need to understand is this:

Habits don't always exist in isolation.

So what you might find is that dealing with your problem habit is not as simple as you think.

You see; Habits can develop out of other existing behaviour.

And just like Rabbits; habits can breed habits.

If one bad habit develops out of another, then it just becomes more complicated.

I liken this process to a “Spiders Web”.

A Spiders Web is created when we have different habits which connect together and support each other.

When it is like this, it can be very difficult to know where to begin and what to do for the best.

The best thing to do is to start somewhere and see what happens. If it is the wrong place, then learn from the experience and start on another.

You will soon find out whether this is something that you are able to do on your own, or whether you need to find some help with it.

You know that you have found the right help and that you are doing the right things; when you begin to get the right results.

> Later there is going to be a chapter on “Symptom Solutioning” and this will help you understand why so many people do the wrong things when they try to deal with a problem.

So what do I want you to take away from this chapter?

Habits exists for all sorts of reasons and purposes.

A habit can be a:

Change agent.
Tolerance tool.
Survival tool.
Relationship tool.
Stress tool. Etc.

A habit has no emotions. It will allow itself to be put to any purpose whether it is good or bad.

As people, we have the ability to modify and change habits, remove them and create new ones.

As we do so; we can change, modify and improve:

Your Life Profile.

At the beginning of every day:

You have the opportunity to write the Life Profile you want to have; you are not stuck with the one that you currently have.

Get into the habit of Living a Better Life and Improving Your Life Profile.

CHAPTER 15

The Role Of Relationships In Your Problem

There are many different and good books about Relationships.

So I am not going to go into all the different aspects of relationships that there are.

Instead; what I am going to focus on are the aspects that I want to highlight as being relevant and appropriate to Persistent Weight Problems.

In a sense I am going to point out:

"The Tips Of Iceberg's"

Those things that are visible above the surface but that may have a lot hidden beneath; that may be contributing to the development and maintenance of someone's problem with their weight.

All of us, without exception, have relationships with People and Things.

Some of us have fewer than we want and some of us have more than we want.

All of us, at some time or another, don't have the Right Types of relationships.

Sometimes it's family relationships that are the problem and other times it is friendships that are a problem.

Sometimes it's work related relationships that are the problem.

Sometimes we are lonely and at other times we long for solitude.

Sometimes we want physical closeness and at other times we want emotional connections.

Sometimes we just want the recognition from another person that we exists. And that we have not become insignificant to the world. And a simple conversation with another human being can make a difference to us.

All of us Want and Need something from another person, at one time or another!

This requires Interactions at a personal level.

In my experience where there are significant problems; such as a weight problem. Then there is always a problem, or problems, with relationships around somewhere.

If there is a family then it is not unusual for the Mother to become a "Dogs Body" and have to give up their own identity and personal activities for the family.

Sometimes this role is undertaken by the Father.

Sometimes this role is undertaken by another member of the family or even a friend.

> Sacrifice and Compromise in relationships can cause serious problems at times. Especially when it goes too far or goes on for too long.

I have worked with a number of people who have found themselves in this type of situation.

Eventually they begin to lose "Themselves" in the process of looking after and looking out for others.

Their own personal rewards in life continually get put to the back of their priority list. And eventually all of this becomes normal.

Their Needs don't really count or matter and eventually they only matter for what they can do for others. They become Facilitators of other people's lives but not their own.

Over time Resentment creeps in to the best of relationships where someone isn't being sufficiently valued; or doesn't feel as if they are.

Resentment is one of those things that can fester over time and begin to creep into other areas of life and affect other aspects of life.

Aspects such as Sex, Closeness, Trust, Confidence, Self-Esteem and Self-Worth can all be affected.

So a "Giving Person" can find themselves in a relationship where there is too little in the relationship for them. How do they then begin to deal with that?

This then brings us to Love.

Things can get terribly complicated by Love and Affection.

Love of children, love of parents, love of partner, love of position, love of pets, love of home, etc.

How do we deal with things when Love and Affection complicate a problem?

Then there is Guilt.

Oh, we can feel terribly guilty when we have negative thoughts about our loved ones.

And how do we handle those guilty feelings?

Then there may be the feelings that we have when we are not getting enough Attention.

> Well we are part of this relationship and we should be treated like a Valued person; shouldn't we?

Do you feel like you are asking the other person to choose between you and your children; or their children; or their sick or old parent?

The reality is that NO-ONE is immune to Relationships; Good ones or Bad ones.

Of course there are the people who will tell you that:

"It doesn't matter"

That there is:

"Nothing Wrong!"

But what is the costs to them of Burying or Disconnecting from their Feelings and their Needs?

And then there are the Selfish Ones.

I am talking about the Truly Selfish Ones.

Not the ones who are being Bullied and told that they are Selfish; as they are punished in some way.

I am talking about the ones who are likely to be on the other side of this equation.

The ones where No-one and Nothing that they have is good enough.

These are the people who can so easily cause harm to others and also to themselves; if they have sufficient self-awareness.

What do you do if you find yourself on the wrong side of a selfish relationship?

Then there are those who are simply: Just Cruel.

Those who relish and enjoy the pain and suffering of others.

Those who make it a point to destroy relationships, ruin friendships, destroy confidence, kill happiness and ruin other people's lives.

Relationships can give us happiness and they can make us unhappy as a result of what we do and what we expect or want from them.

However; there is a secret with relationships, regardless of whether the relationships are good or bad.

The secret is:

> That we often have more control in any Relationship situation than we understand or than we can think is permitted to us.

So many times I have had to help people to manage their relationships in different ways as part of the process of helping them resolve, improve and better manage other life problems; such as their weight.

Let's not pretend that Relationships are easy all the time or that there are easy fixes for all relationship problems. Because there are not.

Sometimes it comes down to hard choices and difficult courses of action.

That old saying:

> You can choose your friends but you cannot choose your family is true.
>
> However; you can choose how you want to manage both of these and the level and type of involvement that you want to have.

The process of Managing Relationships can often begin from the position of:

"Being On The Back Foot".

That is to say that you are out of position, off-balance, really down, tired out, worn out, completely confused, befuddled, under resourced, beaten-up, scared and afraid, desperate, lonely, etc.

The reality is that we all have to begin from wherever we are at; wherever that may be.

Because wherever we are at, is it:

The Starting Point!

Relationships, or the absence of Relationships, will form Chapters in Your Life Profile.

Many of our relationships also have Habitual parts to them. Some of these will be beneficial and some may not be.

With each Relationship we have the choices of:

- Continuing to write the same things into our Life Profiles.
- Changing what we write.
- Deciding to stop writing that chapter.
- To begin writing another chapter; that tells our story in a different way.

So what do I want you to take away from this chapter?

Avoid The Knee Jerk Nuclear Option!

The reality is that relationships do break-up.

As part of fixing a long term weight problem we need to address Influencing Factors and relationships are Influencing Factors.

I normally like to try and take the Steam out of a situation and bring some long term thinking and clarity into the situation. Before anyone makes any drastic long term decisions; such as to end a marriage, move home, change locations or give up a career.

This is not always possible but it usually works.

> By delaying critical life decisions until such time as we can see them clearly and without built up resentment; we can generally make better ones.

When someone has put up with difficulties in a relationship for a long time, and things have come to a head; probably because the weight problem has escalated, they often feel compelled to take drastic action.

In my experience the drastic action can often be the wrong action, at the wrong time, for the wrong reasons.

> Don't think that any significant relationships that you have (or don't have) are not influencing your behaviours. They will be!

CHAPTER 16

The Role Of "A Lack of Understanding" In Your Problem

A large part of what this book is attempting to do; is to help you understand a weight problem by taking an alternative view.

I am trying to move your thinking away from the conventional and easy approach that people usually take.

> The "Easy Thing" to do with a weight problem is to focus on a diet and exercise programme.
>
> The "Hard Thing" to do is to move away from this position; and look at the things that are behind and driving a weight problem forwards; and keeping it going.

One of the problems with the "Hard Thing" is that, most of the time, the person with the weight problem doesn't actually understand the different Human Dynamics that are part of their problem and which are influencing them.

In effect; what they have is a lack of Understanding and a lack of Comprehension about the problem itself. And about what's actually required to sort it out properly.

This is not their fault and it is not a wilful thing; it is just the reality of the structure of the problem itself.

The lack of Understanding and the lack of Comprehension occurs, in a large part, because of the way that the problem itself evolves.

Weight problems normally evolve over time; and things associated with a weight problem generally happen gradually and at a slow pace.

Weight problems and the associated issues that develop; integrate and become blended together over a period of months, years and decades.

The progression is slow; and because it is slow the person misses it.

> Because of the slow progression of the problem; they lack the perspective to see the real differences between how life Is now and how life Was before.
>
> So as they are losing something; they fail to see it going and to understand the full impact of losing it.

To be able to remedy the weight problem we need to address this process, and to do so, we need to go through a New Learning Process.

Some of this involves filling in all the gaps from your life experiences and understandings that exist, and which affects your Lifestyle Management.

Much of the work that is required would be considered to be Experiential Learning.

Experiential learning is Learning by Doing and Experiencing; while having someone to guide you.

To show you how effective this process is:

> Your weight problem developed as a result of this process!
>
> It just happens that it went wrong.

In order to get to where you are:

> You Experimented and learned and adapted your behaviours.

We use this same process to Evolve the problem into a Positive Outcome; rather than the Negative Outcome that you have.

This can be a difficult thing to facilitate with another person and I developed the Human Dynamics Matrix and other tools to help me with this process.

It helps both the facilitator and the person with the problem to understand the different Human Dynamics which are involved and that need to be worked with.

It helps us to see things with the Correct Perspective and Understanding, so that we can then deal with them effectively.

I am using The Dieters Scale© in this book to begin to help you see things differently. Is it working?

So what do I want you to take away from this chapter?

Many problems develop because of the lack of the right type of education, life skills and structures.

Weight problems are the same!

> We use what we have to understand and work with life problems and life challenges that we encounter.
>
> And if we don't have what we need; then we try to find it elsewhere or adapt and use what we do have.

Somehow or other those gaps in someone's Life Education, need to be filled in with the right type of Education and Information.

The greater the degree of your Weight Problem, and the Associated and Related Problems; the greater the time and Experiential Work that will be required for the restructuring of the framework of your life.

> If the degree of your problems falls into the Green Zone, then this should take less time and have less difficulties attached to them than someone whose problems fall into the Amber Zone.
>
> If the degree of your problems falls into the Amber Zone or Red Zone then this will take more time than the person who falls into the Green Zone.

Chapter 17

The Role Of Symptom Solutioning In Your Problem

The reality is that Persistent Weight Problems take time to develop and there are processes that allow and cause it to happen.

No-one just wakes up one morning to find that they have a persistent weight problem.

The might wake up to the realisation that they have a weight problem and the scale of it; but the problem would have been there for some time.

If your weight problem falls into the Green Zone of the Dieters Scale, then it will have developed to a different Degree than someone whose weight problem falls into the Amber or Red Zones.

In effect; you are all travelling along the same Weight Spectrum but you are at different places on it.

If you carry on doing what you are doing; where will it take you?

Usually it will take you further down the road from where you are and in the direction that you are heading.

So what may be contributing to your problem and undermining your efforts; without you realising it?

The role of "Symptom Solutioning" in the development and maintenance of your problem.

Symptom Solutioning© is a process of dealing with the consequences of problems, in isolation or without regard to the things which are actually causing the problems.

And repeating this process with new and ongoing problems.

As a result of doing this; over time, you lose touch with the real problems and become more focused on dealing with the consequences.

Symptom Solutioning also involves distracting people away from their life problems and dissatisfactions. By claiming that you can provide them with something which helps them achieve the good things that they desire, in a simple and easy way.

This distraction process often involves fantasy thinking and expectations. And if you look at Television any day of the week you will see hundreds of examples of this in commercials for all sorts of products and services.

Persistent Weight problems are a classical example of Symptom Solutioning and the consequences of Symptom Solutioning.

> A typical diet class treats the Symptom – Being overweight. Yo-Yo dieting is the consequence of constantly trying to deal with the Symptom of the weight problem – Being fat.

Let's look at Diet Clubs, for example:

What does the script for virtually all diets say:

You are going to lose (X) weight over (Y) weeks!

And how often does someone then approach the diet with the expectations that they will be able to lose (X) weight over (Y) weeks; and then be able to keep it going?

And what other Expectations are they also bringing into the dieting process?

A lot more!

For example:

Once I have lost that weight I will be able to...

As a result of these expectations you are actually expecting the dieting process to Facilitate Results that the solution cannot provide; but which are often being sold to you through the marketing for these products.

For example:

How often do you see a diet being marketed with slim and attractive people?

How often are these people shown as being Confident, Happy, Self-Assured and Desirable; and living a lifestyle that you really want?

All the time!

This is because this is what we want to see and this is what we really want to achieve from the dieting process.

We want to have, and live, a Better Quality of Life!

> So Implicitly they show you that you can achieve this by using their products and services.

If they showed you the real success rate from their dieting solutions over a period of years; you would probably not buy it.

Diet classes run with very high failure rates and always welcome you back.

And you find that once a diet has run its course and numbers are falling off; they revamp it and begin marketing it again using words like:

- New!
- More effective.
- New formula.
- Eat more of what you like.
- Easier.
- And they often include Scientific Sounding claims.

How many of the people who are providing diets have taken the time to understand the "True Nature" of a real diet problem?

Don't confuse the ability to sell diets with understanding a weight problem. They are not the same thing.

Failing to understand the real nature and structure of the problem that you are dealing with; and instead treating the consequences, is doing the following:

> It's making you feel temporarily better and this can be like a Placebo Effect.
>
> With a Placebo; It doesn't do you any real good, unless you think that it does; but it is meant to do you no real harm.

We could look at the practices of most of the diet industry in this way.

However; my view is that many people are harmed by the Consequential Effect/Affect of repeated dieting; which fails to deliver on the promises it makes through its advertising and the general Persona that it develops for the different brands.

> The failure to deliver not only shows in someone's weight; it is also experienced through other areas of their lives.

The truth is that Persistent Weight Problems require a good dose of reality and to be grounded in reality for them to be effective long term.

Reality however; is both sweet and sour. And not many people like taking both of these if they are offered a choice.

Most people want the sweet.

> Most people are so sensitive to their weight problem that they cannot handle a good dose of reality and being grounded in reality.
>
> So this then sets-up the cycle for Symptom Solutioning to continue and grow.

The truth is that lots of people can help you to lose weight in the short term. What everyone struggles with is making it past the short term and turning it into a longer term sustainable result.

So everyone focuses on the short term.

- The seller and provider of the diet.
- The use of the diet.
- The seller of consumable products.
- The user of the consumable products.

This bias towards short term thinking, short term results and small amounts of effort; just pushes people more towards Symptom Solutioning and away from the more difficult long term successful solution that they really want and need.

> If the solution you are applying to the problem cannot resolve that problem; then there is no way that it can work other than through luck!

Why rely on luck when you can rely on solutions that have been developed to deal with the problems in the right ways.

Life Improvement Programmes Focused On Weight

With my Life Improvement Programmes and the other work that I do; we work with reality from the start.

We have to or we just end up going in the wrong direction and wasting time.

When things are done in the right way and with the right expectations, I find that people with persistent weight problems can and do handle it well.

The structure of the Programmes means that we are in a comfortable position to deal with difficult life issues.

Our structure also helps those who are on the programmes to learn and develop new skills and new ways of dealing with difficult and complicated issues.

Persistent Weight problems are really Lifestyle Management Problems.

This is what we work with as part of a Life Improvement Programme – How to manage our Lifestyles better so that we can achieve the Life that we want and become free of the tyranny and pressures of dieting and weight control.

So what do I want you to take away from this chapter?

As you move into different Zones on The Dieters Scale©, problems will increase in size and complexity.

All problems have a structure and that structure can be understood.

All solutions have a structure and that structure can be understood.

To remedy complex problems you need to understand and work with the Components of the problem and the Components of the solution.

Problems are successfully resolved, improved and managed, when we have a good fit between the structure of the problem and the structure of the solution.

It becomes as simple as Square Pegs and Rounds Holes.

The worse the fit, the more reliant we become on luck.

Perhaps more diets should be called:

The Lucky Diet.

CHAPTER 18

The Role Of Food In Your Problem

Have you ever heard someone with a weight problem say:

"An alcoholic can stop drinking
but I can't stop eating or I will die!"

If you haven't heard this particular saying then you may have heard of other sayings that justify someone's eating behaviour.

Basically what many people are saying is:

That they are Powerless in the presence of food.

Part of the problem which we have, as Imperfect People, is that we want things to be simple and easy.

If we can Easily and Simply avoid the Responsibility for the Consequences of our Dietary Practices, and for the Food that we have Consumed; then we will happily do so.

"I'm not taking the responsibility for eating that Food; it's the Foods fault!

Yep! That's food for you; it jumped straight off that plate and into your mouth. Then it forced your mouth to chew on it, and then you were forced to swallow it and repeat this until all the food was gone.

We have just made a fantastic discovery to explain weight problems:

"Ninja Food"

The reality is that "Ninja Food" just does not exist.

But food can be a powerful and seductive force.

The reality is that Food serves many different purposes other than the basic requirement for nourishment.

In different cultures the preparation, serving and eating of food has cultural and social implications.

We can respect all of these and we can still take responsibility for what we consume.

"I'm Powerless in the face of Food"

There are some who say that they are Powerless when they see or have to look at food.

The reality is that at some point, if you want to be treated as an Adult, then you have to behave like an Adult and show some Restraint.

If you are never going to show Restraint but you want to continue to be treated as a Responsible Adult; then you create a Paradox.

The Paradox you create is the:

I'm an Adult and I want to be treated as an Adult.

BUT

When it comes to my behaviour with Food and the consequences of my behaviour with Food; I can't be held to be a Responsible Adult – Paradox.

Now if you don't want to be a Responsible Adult with Food then other things can happen.

Many years ago FAT PEOPLE who could not help themselves and who developed health problems because of their weight were offered a great solution.

They could have their jaws WIRED SHUT!

All their teeth would be wired and then their teeth would be wired shut so that they could not eat anything because they could not open their mouths.

However; these Adults "who could not help themselves" would do things like:

- Use pliers and cut away the wire when they wanted to eat.
- Liquidise high calorie food, such as chocolate, so that they could pour it through the wire.

And what of those who left the jaw wiring in place and who lost weight; do you think that they continued at that weight when the wiring was finally removed?

Our modern equivalent of this is the Stomach Balloon, the Gastric Band, the Stomach Reduction and other things which are all trying to do the same thing:

> Give the Adult who Can't be Responsible for their own behaviour an easy way to deal with the consequences of their own behaviour.

And those who are having these procedures are demonstrating the same outcomes as those who had their jaws wired shut.

Questions that we should be asking ourselves are:

> Given the increase in the number of people who are having problems with their weight; will we reach a point where they begin to be treated as Disabled People?
>
> Will we reach a point where doctors can determine that the person is "Incapable" and therefore they need to be treated without their consent; for the common good and for their own protection?

Not pleasant thoughts but with about 33% of adults in North America being classified as obese; where do you think this thing is going?

The power to change this is in the hands of the people with the problem; and it is only the people who can change this. Politicians can't!

> The problem isn't the food. The problem is the choices that we make and the actions that we take.

One of the problems with food today is that it is so easily available and so easily stored and moved around.

Food has moved into new areas of life and new types of food have been created.

Portable food has never previously been available like it is today.

The problem for someone with a food problem is often one of convenience.

All they have to do is reach out and they can have some food.

When you have reached a point in your life where you are using food in the wrong ways, and you are not exercising the right choices.

Then quick and easy access to the thing which you are misusing just makes life more difficult.

And it makes managing the problem more difficult.

All it takes to being making long term effective change is:

One Positive Action at a time!

Food offers all of us a lot of Positives. So use and enjoy the Positives.

- Food is there to be enjoyed; so enjoy it.
- Food is there to nourish us; so nourish yourself.
- Food is there to celebrate with; so celebrate.
- Food is there to be appreciated; so appreciate it.

I don't see many people being held down and being forced fed food. In fact; I don't see it ever!

However; you will see people holding themselves down and force feeding themselves!

In reality; most of us, most of the time, have a choice about what we consume, ingest or allow into our bodies.

You can exercise a Pro-Active choice that will benefit you long term; or a Negative choice that will hurt you.

Which do you want to do?

People's bodies are not Consequential Vessels; and they Don't have to behave as if they are.

What this means is that you are not a bystander waiting for people and events to happen to you.

You can become the victim of your own long term behaviour if you want too; or you can Choose Not to be a victim.

The reality for everyone with a Weight problem is:

> That you have more control over this thing than you may care to admit to yourself or than you know.

In fact what is happening to you, that you don't like, is being driven, controlled and managed; largely or wholly by you!

This is the real level of control that you have; even if you do not realise that this is the case.

What I am interested in is helping you to exercise that control in another way.

Let's turn this thing into a Positive rather than a Negative.

If you don't believe this then let me ask you another question:

> Could this problem have occurred without you?

Are You in charge or is the Food in charge of you?

Simple questions show that you are actually acting in ways that puts you in front of the food.

- When you go shopping; who actually agrees the food and who actually puts the food in the trolley?
- Who buys the food?
- Who takes the food home?
- Who cares for and looks after the food?
- Who prepares the food?
- Who puts the food on the plate?
- Who eat the food?

You see:

- Food has no Will.
- Food has no Speech.
- Food doesn't follow us home from the store.
- Food doesn't go out and buy People; People go out and buy food.
- Food doesn't grow people; People grow food.
- Food doesn't abuse People; People abuse food.

Food is Passive and We can put food to any purpose that we want. Good or Bad.

What choices do you want to make today?

So what do I want you to take away from this chapter?

Let's imagine that we were to apply the Dieters Scale© to all the food and other items that you buy and consume.

And if all the items that You were OK with, were put into the Green Zone. What would go into the Green Zone?

If all the items that you had a medium level problem with were put into the Amber Zone. What would go into the Amber Zone?

And then if we put all the items that you had a high level problem with in the Red Zone. What would go into the Red Zone?

This simple process would show you the Zones that your food falls into and also the difficulties that you have with the foods that you are buying and eating.

It will also show you which Zones your eating habits are occupying and give you an idea of how much time your spending in each Zone.

> To do this properly you need to think in terms of your Normal Consumption. Not during a good period but during a Normal Period of time.

The problem isn't **just** the food. The problem is the choices that we make and the actions that we take.

CHAPTER 19

The Role Of "Processed" Foods In Your Problem

I have talked about the Role of Food generally in relation to a Weight Problem.

Now I want to introduce some other aspects that are not normally talked about when we talk about weight problems.

I thought that it was worthwhile including a chapter on Processed Foods.

I want to take a different view of this so:

> What do I mean when I talk about Processed Foods?

I am going to break Processed Foods down into two distinct areas:

1. Processing to Produce and Create Foods.

2. Processing Out the bodies Normal Processing of and Management of Foods.

What we need to understand is: That unless a Food has a component in it; which is toxic or in some way immediately harmful to us:

- That Food related problems can take a long time to materialise.

- Then a long time to become recognised.
- Then a long time to become properly understood.
- And then finally, a long time to get dealt with.

When it comes to food, weight problems and Human Health; the type of question that I ask myself is:

> Are we able to see the problem with the broader and larger scale view required to properly understand it?

I think that in reality; the questions related to these issues are beyond the normal person.

I personally would say that these questions are also beyond our current Governments and the various organisations and groups who control and influence the food industry.

> What I see happening are Responses to obvious problems in the Food Industry, in as simple and easy a manner as is possible.

In effect; The global food industry and those who Police it on our behalf; are caught up in the process of Symptom Solutioning.

They are working with the simple and easy problems and the consequences of other problems; but they are not dealing with the fundamental problems and issues which would make a long term difference.

To change this would require longer term thinking and actions of a type that people who are focused on short term results are not prepared or able to do.

So I think that we are stuck with what we have and that these various Governments and Organisations who control and Police Global Food will respond from crisis to crisis.

> So how does this effect the common man?
>
> And what can we do to reduce the likelihood that we will suffer longer term consequences from the foods and other items that we consume and are exposed too?

What we can do is to try and be more informed and be more pro-active in the actions that we take which involves food.

So let's focus on my two points.

1. Processing to Produce and Create Foods.

2. Processing Out the bodies Normal Processing of and Management of Foods.

And let's deal with the first one.

Processing to Produce and Create Foods.

We have a lot more people on the planet than we had 200 years ago.

During the last 200 years many things have changed.

- New food production practices have been introduced and old ones phased out.
- A faster and easier to service global food market has developed.
- The preservation of foods through the introduction of naturally derived and man-made chemicals has dramatically increased.
- Out of season produce is readily available.
- Preserved, Tinned, bottled, vacuum packed, eradiated and disguised food stuffs have increased and become Normal.
- There has been the development of new classes of Foods that are labelled as "Healthy".
- As Weight problems have grown, so has the number and types of products produced by the Food Industry to deal with this problem.

In amongst all of this is the reality that:

> People need to be fed.
>
> And to keep them healthy, they need nourishing and nutritious foods at an affordable price

This simple process creates Global Dynamics and Tensions which involves Governments,

Businesses, Speculators, Banks, Financial Institutions and Major Supermarkets.

Because of the supply chain, the manufacturing base and the Consumption base; we are all part of this process one way or another and we are all effected by it one way or another.

At the Grass Roots Level we Effect this process through our Consumption, Purchasing and Use.

Most of us think we are Passive Consumers and that we cannot influence things long term. But the truth is:

> Stores don't stock items for long that do not sell!

Ultimately the Global Food and Produce Market is about suppliers needing to find Customers for their goods.

In this search they will look for different ways to replace expensive ingredients with cheaper ingredients.

Formulas for Foods and Produce will be changed, improved and Adulterated.

New chemicals, additives, mixtures, recipes and ingredients will be used.

And they will search out new markets and new applications for the Food and Food related items that they have to sell.

Much of this will be done on the basis of Trust and the Belief that our Governments and the many different organisations involved in the production and distribution of foods; have our best interest at the heart of what they do.

In reality some will and some won't.

I think the global problems that we are experiencing with increasing Obesity is a result of Governments, and the Institutions of Governments, failing to understand what they are dealing with in the global food industries.

And also it is a failure on their part to sufficiently protect their populations that it is their duty to protect.

There are many current practices; such as pumping water and additives into food, which should be curtailed and stopped.

Why should people be paying for water which has been forced into meat?

This is the background which takes me on to my next point and the point that is of most relevance to those with persistent weight problems.

Processing Out; the bodies Normal Processing of and Management of Foods.

I think that hidden within some of the food manufacturing and production that occurs:

> We have Consequential Processes which adversely effects the body.

In effect; what these processes of manufacturing and production are doing is:

> Removing and By-Passing many of the Normal Inhibitors to Excess Weight Gain, that Nature has given us.

And when you do this; you get Unintended Consequences!

We know about the increase in Weight Problems but what about all the other problems that are increasing in numbers; Like Diabetes?

> When we By-Pass and Remove the body's natural inhibitors, we can begin to change the speed at which things happen, and we can begin to change the scale at which things can happen.

So what are the types of processes which are causing these Consequential Effects on people?

If someone gave you 2 lb's (1 kilo) of sugar in a bag and told you to eat that over the next week or so: Would you do so?

If someone gave you 5 apples a day and told you that you have to eat them all; because tomorrow and every other day after that, you will have 5 more pieces of fruit to eat: would you do so?

If someone gave you 2 pints (I litre) of vegetable oil and told you to drink that over the following couple of weeks: Would you do so?

If someone gave you 2 lb's (1 kilo) of hard white, neutral fat and told you to eat that over the coming couple of weeks: Would you do so?

If someone gave you 2 lb's (1 kilo) of different fillers and bulking agents and told you to eat that over the next couple of weeks: Would you do so?

For most people the answers would be NO!

> What we have been able to do with foods through the manufacturing process; is to present foods to you in new ways; so that you are unaware of what you are actually consuming within the foods.

The Food Industry has become better at the use of Flavourings and Colourings. And as a result we can make more Foods appear to be better than they are or to be something that they are not.

Let's take something simple and see how this is being treated.

Let's take: Fruit.

Most of us would agree that Fruit is a healthy food and that consuming fruit must be a healthy activity.

By the normal way of things we consume fruit as a whole item. We eat an apple, a pear or a banana.

Because of our physiology there are Natural Limits on our ability to consume and digest fruit.

So if I was to give you five items of fruit a day (apple, pears, bananas) and I was to ask you to eat them while you ate your normal meals; would you be able to do so?

For most people the answer would be No.

Our physiology gets in the way and you would get put off by the time and effort required for eating the fruit.

However; If I said to you that I was going to turn the fruit into a healthy fruit drink, that would give you your nutrients and vitamins for the day:

> Would you then be able to consume five items of fruit turned into a tasty healthy drink that was good for you?

For most people the answer would be yes!

And this process would be By-Passing your Natural

physiological processes and the limits this imposes.

Of course you may not like fruit. But when it is converted into a tasty healthy drink; you can be convinced that it is good for you and drink it.

Also we can add flavourings and other ingredients to the fruit drink which was harder to do when it was whole.

The point is that if you have to sit down and physically eat five items of fruit a day; this has an effect upon your digestive system.

Your body has to process all the solid food in order to get to the ingredients which are actually in the fruit.

You can't access the sugars until you have physically digested the fruit; and this would take time and the process of accessing the sugars would be slowed down.

However; when we put the fruit into a drink and tell someone that it is healthy: What we have actually done is:

> Remove and By-Passed many of the Normal Inhibitors to Excess Weight Gain, that Nature has given us.

Your body no longer needs to process the solid fruit to get to the sugars. So it's faster.

You no longer have to process the roughage in the

same way through your digestive system. So you lose that benefit and your body isn't doing that work.

You no longer have to chew through five items of fruit; so that inhibition to consumption and over consumption has been removed.

You see not many people would naturally sit down with any real frequency and consume large quantities of fruit along with other foods.

Put them into a drink and you can begin to do this regularly!

And this is the type of thing which has been done to many items of Food.

Things have been added to them which you would not normally consume in that way, in that quantity, in that frequency or in that format.

We have also had things added to foods that you would never, ever want to eat.

And the more that our food is adulterated in this way; the more normal it becomes for us to eat and consume Foods which are adulterated.

Over time our New Normal becomes the Consumption of adulterated Foods because we now have developed a taste for them and our bodies have become used to processing them.

And in our Life Profiles we have written new chapters which includes adulterated and processed Foods.

So now you can begin to see how this all fits together!

> In many instances; if you knew and saw what went into the production of many popular foods; you would want to know more and you would not want to consume many of the items that you found out more about.
>
> And in a world where we are supposed to have greater access to Information; we are actually becoming more ignorant and uninformed about the Foods that we are consuming.

I think that to begin to effectively deal with the issues created by long term persistent weight problems. That you need to take an approach that is not necessarily that of everyone else.

> In reality you have to take a stand for you!

Normal thinking in so many areas of life is around:

> What do we need to do to alleviate the problem.

It is Not:

> How do we alleviate the problem AND stop it from happening again.

If you wait and rely upon the various Governments, Institutions and those who control the Global Food and Produce markets; to make you healthy.

Well you are going to be waiting for quite some time!

So let me tell you what I personally do with foods.

I am one of those people who reads the labels on many of the items that I purchase.

To be able to understand the different names and numbers which are applied to many of the ingredients which are in much of the food; I would have to do a lot of research, and I find this difficult.

In my view: The food industry doesn't actually want us to be informed enough; so that we can EASILY discriminate between the foods that we purchase and consume.

So this is how I personally handle things.

What I do for a few items is that I accept that this thing has ingredients in it, that I am being told about.

But I am being told about them in such a way that I really don't know and understand what is in them.

Then I decide if I actually want it under those terms at that time.

Sometimes I buy and other times I don't.

This would be things like sweets, cakes and sauces; such as pasta sauce.

I don't buy a lot of this type of thing or consume these items on a daily or regular basis.

With a lot of food items that I buy I try to get them as near to the natural state that they were created in.

This would be things like fruit and vegetables, flour, sugar, breakfast cereals, etc.

I have found that I do need to check the labels on some of these items because it is surprising what can be added without you realising it.

For example fruit can be coated in something to help preserve it and make it look better.

I make a lot of what I eat, so I make my own bread, cakes, fruit pies, quiches, etc.

By doing this I find that I use a lot less sugar, salt and yeast. And I eliminate all the ingredients that have to be put into the foods by the manufacturers because of legislation, to preserve the items and to make them taste better.

I also find that food I make myself is normally better tasting and more satisfying. Most of the time.

I do still buy the occasional shop made donut or home-made cake.

I am not a fan of the over consumption of soft drinks and fizzy drinks and so I don't have these very often.

I usually prefer to drink water, tea, coffee or pure orange juice.

I personally do not drink much alcohol and I will have a drink of alcohol every now and again.

Personally I do not eat Beef. This is a decision that I made over 20-years ago and I have stuck with it. I do eat other meats.

I will try to avoid processed meats but I will have them occasionally. This will be things like sausages.

I don't eat much in the way of prepared sliced meats as more other ingredients are being added to them and I can't see the point of adding them.

I like cheeses and I am happy to eat them but I try to avoid any where things like colouring have been added. Though this is getting more difficult.

I like different types of bread and I love home-made pizza's (the base has to be home-made). I make most of the bread that I eat.

I like fish and I probably eat more fish than meat.

I try to avoid most foods where colourings have been added to improve the appearance of the food; such as can happen with cheese and fish.

I avoid too much in the way of sauces and coatings which have been added to foods. I prefer to taste the food and not the sauces.

I do eat out. I rarely have a Take-Away meal. And I generally prefer simple but well cooked food.

So my diet is not too restrictive and I eat a broad range of foods.

If I am not happy with something about a food or a retailer; then I will change my choice and the retailer.

I don't have a weight problem but I know that when I eat certain foods too often, that I can begin to gain weight. When I do begin to gain weight, I then cut these foods out or reduce them in my diet.

All of this is part of my Lifestyle Management.

> I take an active part in the selection of the foods that I consume.
>
> I take responsibility when I consume something that may not be great but that I feel like eating at that time.
>
> If I see that I am gaining weight, then I take an active part in dealing with that problem. I take the step of altering my diet and my lifestyle.

We can't be 100% in control of all the Foods that we consume. But we can be in control of enough of it to make a long term difference to the quality of our lives and our health.

So what do I want you to take away from this chapter?

Is any part of your weight problem being caused by behaviour or the consumption of foods which assist in:

> The Removing and By-Passing of the Normal Inhibitors to Excess Weight Gain, that Nature has given us.

If you are; then you may experience Unintended Consequences.

We know about Weight Problems but what about all the other problems that are increasing in numbers; Like Diabetes?

> When we By-Pass and Remove the body's natural inhibitors, we can begin to change the speed at which things happen and we can begin to change the scale at which things can happen.

Type 2 Diabetes can often be brought under control and resolved by good dietary practices, exercise and better Lifestyle Management.

Note
Many of the new fast fixes such as pills that help you to stop absorbing all the fat from the foods that you eat are, it would seem, simply attempting to put back some of the natural inhibitors that food processing has removed. This is just more Symptom Solutioning and it doesn't fix the problem.

Chapter 20

The Role Of Exercise In Your Problem

Physical activity of certain types is necessary to human health. Any reasonable person would agree with this.

As our lifestyles have changed, we have reduced and ceased much of the physical activity that we need to do to keep us fit and healthy.

To help combat these changes to our lives, Planned and Structured Physical Activities have been developed to help us; and we call these Exercises.

Some forms of exercise have evolved beyond that required for physical health and these have become specialisations. Many of those specialisations develop to include Social Functions.

For example; swimming, football, golf and going to the gym involve social exercising and socialising.

What all exercise has in common is that our bodies and our minds are challenged by activities.

The role of exercise in your problem.

I am an advocate of keeping fit and healthy without going to extremes.

I know and understand the benefits of working out and keeping fit as I have done so all my life.

There are obvious benefits to keeping fit and there are less obvious benefits.

Let's see how these benefits may Effect and Affect us; and benefit someone with a weight problem.

First let's clarify why I am using Effect and Affect.

> **Effect** is a Result or Consequence. Something which we bring about, accomplish, cause to exist or occur.
>
> Normally we need to Do something or Not Do something for this to happen.
>
> So doing exercise allows us to create a Result or produce a Consequence.
>
> For example; getting and maintaining a level of fitness would be the Effect.
>
> **Affect** is a Feeling or Emotion. Something which we can experience within our mind and our body as a consequence or result of other actions.
>
> So when we become fit, we can experience the Affect of Feeling Better about ourselves.
>
> The Affect of Feeling more confidence and thinking that we look better.

Basically: What all this means is that Actions can lead to Feelings and Emotions; and Feelings and Emotions can lead to Actions.

So this process is a fundamental part of what makes us tick and it gives us a Formula to use!

- Emotions & Feelings can produce Actions.
- Actions can produce Emotions & Feelings.

This simple formula gives us a way to begin to influence and change things and to understand how our own problems with our weight comes about over time.

I think that most people tend to think of exercise as:

"Keeping or Getting Fit"

The reality is that Getting and Keeping Fit is just one purpose for exercise; there are others.

The mental discipline that it helps to create can be very beneficial to those with persistent weight problems.

The good feelings that you experience when you have completed a workout make it worthwhile.

The satisfaction you feel when you have worked out; even though you really didn't feel like it when you started the workout.

It can be very useful when you are stressed.

Keeping fit when you are stressed helps to avoid and reduce stress related problems. And it helps to better manage longer terms problems that can effect our physiology; such as tension.

So in reality there are Mental, Physical and Emotional benefits to be had from appropriate exercise. Let's call these Your Inner World Benefits.

And there are Lifestyle Benefits to be had from appropriate exercise. Let's call these Your Outer World Benefits.

Like many other things; Exercise has also been presented as a Quick Fix solution to weight problems.

How often have you heard things like:

- Burn that excess fat off through doing...
- Increase your metabolic rate and target those fat cells.

I can see the attraction of this approach to people who want to lose weight and look better quickly.

However there is a flaw with this approach.

It introduces the belief that you can immediately effect your weight by doing exercise and that this has burned off fat and calories.

But the reality of how the body works suggest that this is not going to happen the way that you may be being sold it.

According to my current understanding of Human Physiology these attempts at targeting the "Unwanted " and "Overweight Fat" and the "Bloated Fat Cells" through exercise are unproven and unlikely.

And the simple truth is; that if all this stuff was that simple and easy, then it would be really simple for the people who market these things to prove it; again and again.

> It would be as simple as 10 overweight people in at one end of the process and 8 slim people out at the other!
>
> And if it was that simple and easy then would we really have so many overweight people?
>
> Because I am sure that many of them would use this simple easy way, if it was real.

In reality it takes time and concentrated effort for the physical accumulation of muscle and for the reduction in bloated fat cells.

It is possible to Misused Exercise in the same way that any other form of behaviour can be misused.

People can and do take exercise to extremes, where they Over-Do the amount, type and frequency of the exercise that they are doing.

Then there are the people who go to the other extreme. Those who never do anything that may resemble exercise. In fact; they are Appalled by the very thought of any exercise.

Regardless of your current views on exercise:

> Some form of physical activity which challenges your body in appropriate ways is essential for physical, mental and emotional health.

So why should someone with a Persistent Weight Problem; have any interest in this at all?

- After all: Exercise is just so much hot air, sweat, hard work, inconvenience, etc.

Maybe so: But let's take another look at the Formula that I said can help us to Influence and Change things.

- Emotions & Feelings can produce Actions.
- Actions can produce Emotions & Feelings.

If you can; now relate this to your Habits with Food?

- Do you ever respond differently to food as a result of how you feel?

- Do you ever feel better as a result of preparing, getting or eating food?

The answer should be Yes; of course you do!

> In all the Actions and Re-Actions that we have to different things; the body is involved.

So Nature has given us all this wonderful free gift of a body.

It has given us the Free Will to use it as we want.

The question that you face is:

- How do you want to use yours?

Do you want to use it in a Pro-Active way and Influence your life?

Do you want to use it in a Re-Active way and be influenced and controlled by whatever you come into contact with?

Either way your body is going to be involved and as you live in your body; you will also be involved.

- Being Pro-Active gives you More Opportunity to Influence things in a Positive and Beneficial way.

- Being Re-Active gives you Less Opportunity to Influence things in a Positive and Beneficial way.

If you want More Opportunity to have the Life that you really want; then you are More Likely to Achieve this by Being Pro-Active.

And this is the simple prize that exist behind the Door of Opportunity called Exercise:

> Exercise lets you begin to be Pro-Active in a simple and easy way that is personal to you.

As a result of the exercise, you begin to influence your emotions and feelings.

And when you are someone with a weight problem; this is important.

So what do people do wrong with exercise that screws things up?

The Wrong Timing!

Ok; so you have gone on a diet. And to burn that fat off quicker you have signed up at the local gym.

Your ticking all the boxes on the Go On A Diet and Get Fit campaign.

And within a short period of time; your struggling.

Earlier in this book I talked about the stress of changing too many things in your life at the same time.

For many people going on a diet and beginning a Get Fit campaign is too much.

All the stuff you are doing is too new. You haven't adjusted. Your body hasn't adjusted and you don't know how to handle it.

So what do I suggest to people when it comes to exercise?

Simple:

You don't have to wait until you are on a diet to begin exercising.

Why not begin doing a little bit of exercise before you actually plan to go on a diet?

Take a few weeks, or better still take a few months, and begin a gradual process of getting and maintaining Being and Feeling fitter.

Too Much, Too Soon!

Getting and Being Fitter does not mean that I want to become an athlete.

And If I play golf, it doesn't mean that I want to become a professional golfer.

It just means that I want to try and enjoy these activities, get some fun out of them, enjoy a degree of challenge and get the benefits of exercise from them.

And yet so many people who go on a diet and exercise programme; Throw Themselves into the process to such a degree that they cannot sustain it.

They do too much, too soon!

On my Life Improvement Programmes I do not encourage people to begin exercising.

In fact I often discourage it.

The reason why I do this is that the person has enough to deal with at that time, without adding anything unnecessary at that time.

In all of this Timing is important.

There will be a time when exercise is appropriate and it can Add To and Compliment what we are doing.

However; there are times when it is Inappropriate and it can Detract From and Complicate what we are doing.

I find that as we move through the process of the Life Improvement Programme; that there is a point at which exercise and addressing the issue of exercise becomes appropriate.

And what I always suggest to someone as a way to begin getting fitter; is walking.

Plain old simple Walking.

Walking is often the easiest form of exercise for someone to do.

They can go as slow as they like, as long as they keep going.

It is easy to gradually increase the pace at which you walk and to vary the pace at which you walk.

It is easy to increase the distance that you walk and you have lots of choice about where and when you walk.

Walking can also be easily introduced into your lifestyle.

Using the stairs rather than the lift. Walking to the shops for small items rather than using the car.

Walking is a simple process that can produce great results that you cannot see but which you benefit from.

The Wrong Type!

I have exercised and chosen to keep fit and active for most of my life.

During this time I have tried many different activities. Some were very strenuous and some were very placid.

I now have a selection of activities which I do regularly.

I swim, I go for walks, I exercise in my gym at home where I cycle and run on the equipment that I have.

So why do I cycle and run on equipment at home rather than go outside?

Simple: I have an injury to my knee which is permanent. If I run and cycle on the roads, the impact causes problems with the injury. If I do this at home I get the exercise, which benefits me, but without the injury problems.

Another reason why I work out at home is convenience. I don't have to travel to a gym, so I save myself all that time and inconvenience.

I can also work out at a time that suits me. It's more convenient.

What we need to understand and accept is that as we move through life our bodies change. They become less subtle, less resilient and we pick up injuries and restrictions due to living life.

So it stands to reason that with all the different types of exercise that are available for us to do; that some Will Suit Us and be Appropriate and some Will Not Suit Us and be Inappropriate.

Also our exercise needs will change as the weight problem changes.

What we really need to do is to apply The Dieters Scale© to the exercises that we are considering doing, so that we can get a proper measurement.

In The Dieters Scale; we have the Green, Amber and Red Zones.

We know that the Green Zone is the easiest and most straightforward of all the Zones.

For the purpose of putting exercise in The Dieters Scale we will use the following guidelines.

- Green would be easy to moderate exercise.
- Amber would be moderate to difficult exercise.
- Red would be difficult to impossible exercise.

Now The Dieters Scale© is personal for you and it is not intended to be used by your local gym.

They would see things in a different way to you and it is you that we are interested in and not your local gym.

So how would we use this?

Let's use walking as a way to understand the process of using The Dieters Scale© for Exercise.

Let's begin with someone who has a weight problem and they are going on a diet.

They want to get fit and we want to see whether they will be able to sustain the exercises that they are planning to do.

Let's assume that when they plan to begin, they are not fit at all.

Green Zone Exercise's

So if someone was to begin exercising using the Green Zone level, what would that look like:

Any form of walking, slow or moderate pace, for up to 1 hour; or 3 miles in distance.

This would be the target that you would aim to be able to maintain your walking at.

You would look to achieve this over a period of say 1-2 months.

This is over and above any walking that you would normally do in your day-to-day life.

You would be Doing this twice a week, with a gap of 2-3 days between each walk and this would become part of your lifestyle.

This level would begin to get you fit, if you were unfit to begin with.

Amber Zone Exercise's

So if someone was to begin exercising using the Amber Zone level, what would that look like:

Any form of walking, moderate to fast pace, for up to 2.5 hours; or 5-6 miles in distance.

This is over and above any walking that you would normally do in your day-to-day life.

Doing this three times a week with a day between each walk.

This level would get you fit and keep you fit; but you would struggle to do it and keep it going if you were not fit to begin with.

You would be Doing this three times a week and this would become part of your lifestyle.

So we can see that if you hadn't gone through the Green Zone process of Getting Fit to begin with.

And you tried to do this as your fitness programme; that you would probably struggle and fail.

> I would NOT suggest that you try this level until you could easily do the Green Zone Level and had done that for several months.

Now let's look at the Red Zone level.

Red Zone Exercise's

So if someone was to begin exercising using the Red Zone level, what would that look like:

Any form of walking, moderate to fast pace, for up to 4 hours; covering 10 miles or more in distance.

This is over and above any walking that you would normally do in your day-to-day life.

Doing this 4-5 times a week or more and this would become part of your lifestyle.

This level would get you fit and keep you fit but you would struggle to do it and keep it going if you were Amber Level fit to begin with.

> So we can see that if you were at the Green Zone Level of fitness to begin with; then you would almost certainly fail if you did a Red Zone level fitness programme.

Let's look at what is going on with the process of getting fit in the different Zones of The Dieters Scale.

As you go up the Dieters Scale, from the Green Zone to the Amber and Red Zones, the level of commitment required to achieve the results increases.

The time required to achieve the results increases.

The energy and level of fitness required to produce the results increases.

Your body has to have the ability to recover from the exercise quickly. Your muscles need to be use to the exercise that they are undertaking to do this.

The amount of your life that is "Occupied" by the activities required to achieve the results increases.

So if we have someone who would struggle to exercise in the Green Zone when they begin a diet and exercise programme; and we put them into the Amber or Red Zone; what outcome would we expect?

- They would struggle.
- Increasing stress.
- Very uncomfortable.
- Injury.
- Hungry.
- Self conscious.
- Etc.

And often the more that the person needs the benefits of exercise, the less able they are to engage with exercise that falls outside of the Green Zone level.

Even when we take our Unfit person and we apply the Green Zone level of exercise to them; they can experience everything in the list above.

It is just part of the process that people go through when they are unfit and they want to get fit.

So; what often happens in the real world?

People who would be appropriate for the Green Zone level go and try and do the Amber and Red Zone exercise level; with the inevitable result:

They fail!

And this keeps the dieting cycle going and the weight problem going.

> What this book and my Life Improvement Programmes are about; is breaking and changing the cycle of events, actions, re-actions and outcomes.
>
> By doing this we help the person live a better life and become a more successful person.
>
> Every person has the ability within themselves to achieve this; what they usually need help with is finding, applying and managing that ability.

Let's look at another myth.

I'm Not Sweating!

One of the Myths of exercise is that you need to sweat. And the more that you sweat; the better the exercise is for you.

In reality we all need to challenge our bodies and this means working them harder.

If we work our bodies hard enough then we sweat.

As well as sweating when we exercise, we also sweat for other reasons.

- We are hot and we need to cool down.
- We are stressed, nervous, etc.

If you are very unfit then you may sweat whenever you do anything physical.

What you need to understand about sweating is this:

> Sweating does not mean that you are exercising correctly or sufficiently.

When I work out I sweat. This is because I am doing a lot of hard work over a short time. I need to sweat to keep my body from getting too hot.

If I go out walking, then for most of the walk I am not sweating. This is because I am exercising but not getting too hot.

If I start walking faster or walking up hills then I am likely to sweat.

So if I do not walk too fast or up hills, then I can have a long walk without sweating.

So I can have what is called a Low Impact Workout.

Low impact workouts give you the benefits of exercise in a low key way.

This level of exercise would be in the Green Zone.

Walking can provide a good low impact workout and this is why I will suggest walking as an exercise.

Don't worry if you are not sweating when you exercise; especially in the beginning.

Sooner or later you will move to a position where you will sweat because you get fitter and you can challenge your body in a more profitable way.

If you have exercised over a long time (months or years) and you don't sweat when you exercise.

Then you may be failing to understand what exercise is; or you may need to increase or vary what you do.

Sweating isn't good or bad; it is just an indicator.

So what do I want you to take away from this chapter?

Physical activity is a requirement for a healthy body, a healthy mind and a healthy lifestyle.

However: The level of physical activity, the type of physical activity and the longevity of physical activity varies from person to person and situation to situation.

It also varies according to what your long term goals are for undertaking the exercise in the first place:

- Are you getting and keeping fit?
- Are you training to be an athlete?

Very few people will get into difficulty with exercise, if they are exercising within the Green Zone level on The Dieters Scale.

The Green Zone level will get you fit and allow you to maintain a fitness level without too much impact on your lifestyle.

You have to get the Timing right for when you introduce exercise or increase exercise.

If the timing is wrong it just puts someone under too much pressure that can then impact other things.

Remember: Exercise is not a very good way of losing weight!

My examples of walking are not recommendations they are to illustrate a concept.

I would not have any problems with recommending the Green Zone level of exercise to any of my friends or family who were looking to get fit.

Exercise, especially before meals, can affect the way that our bodies manage and process the foods that we eat.

We are only just beginning to understand these effects but there are positive results showing that the body handles the food that you consume in a better way after exercise; and it does not have to be prolonged hard exercise.

As a rule of thumb; we should always avoid exercising too soon after we have eaten. And eating too soon after we exercise.

CHAPTER 21

The Role Of "Influencing Factors" In Your Problem

In a previous chapter I looked at the role of relationships in your problem; and I talked about the Tips of the Icebergs of different issues.

What I want to do now is move this closer and look at individual people, and other things which can influence your behaviour, and which may affect you and your persistent weight problem.

I also want to take a glimpse at your relationships with them.

> If we are maintaining too many of the wrong types of relationships with the wrong type of people; then we will suffer a Negative and ongoing Consequence as a result of our interactions with those people.
>
> If we are maintaining the wrong type of relationship with the right type of people; then can we change this to the right type of relationship?

I am not getting into any form of judgement of the people or how they live their lives.

I just want you to begin to take a look at the relationships that you have, in a way that can help you to put your efforts into the ones that help you, rather than hurt you.

In reality; different types of relationships, whether good, bad or indifferent are able to influence us.

Therefore they are Influencing Factors.

And that is what we are interested in – Influencing Factors.

> Many people never actually look at the relationships that they have with their family, friends and work associates in this way.
>
> Other very important Influencing Factors to consider are television, magazines and the Internet.

Because people tend not to look at these Influencing Factors with a critical eye; they fail to see when things are going wrong or that there are issues which need to be addressed.

This happens with both Positive and Negative influencing factors.

> So if we never discriminate between Positive Influencing Factors which help us and make our lives better. And Negative Influencing Factors which can harm us and make our lives worse.
>
> Then we end up with a range of Influencing Factors which we Respond Too, and over which, we are exercising little real Positive Control.
>
> So it's no wonder that things can get messy!

We could use The Dieters Scale© to help us grade these Influencing Factors but I will just touch upon different things so as to get you thinking.

Now I don't know how many people you know and what sort of relationships you have with them. So I am going to lay this out in a general way and you can adjust this for your own personal circumstances.

There are a number of things to think about with Influencing Factors; including:

- How many of them there are.
- Whether they are Positive or Negative.
- How much of our time are we exposed to them.
- How impactful are they on us.
- How dependent are we upon them.
- Do we need to end that relationship/exposure.
- Do we want to keep that relationship and change something about it.
- Are there Passive Influencing Factors which are affecting us that we are not noticing.
- Do we need to find new ones.

I don't expect you to sit down today and sort this out. I would like you to be aware of this and begin to think about it and the role that this plays in your life and with your problem.

If I was working with someone; this is something that we would gradually address over time.

In order to bring this into your awareness; let's see how this could be structured.

When we consider the people that we spend time with and are influenced by; there is a simple question that we want to know.

How Close are they to you?

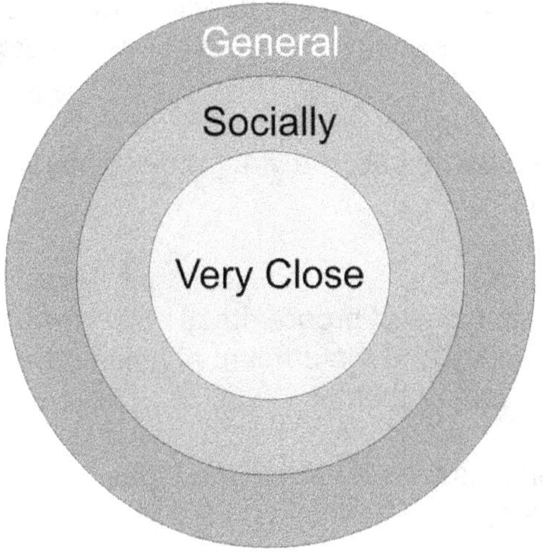

Is this person a friend, work associate, family member or just someone you occasionally run into?

Generally the closer the person is to you, the more difficult it can be to do something about the relationship, if there are problems with it.

The graphic above shows the people who are closest to you as being in the centre of your Circle of Influence.

Then the next layer shows those who you are not very close too; but who form part of your Social Network and who can influence you socially.

The outside layer shows the rest of the contacts that you will have, that can influence you. This layer includes general things like Televisions, Internet, Films and Games.

Now it may be that you don't have many very close people and that your life is very limited. It may be that you are spending most of your time watching the TV.

> Then these become your closest influencing factors.

Where this is the case; the next thing would be to look at the types of programmes you are watching, the frequency and the amount of time that you spend watching them.

This helps us to understand the types of influences that watching TV brings into your life.

So it doesn't matter whether you have a very busy life with lots of people in your life. Or whether you have a very empty life with no people but plenty of distractions.

What matters here is what you actually have and not what you want.

As you begin to allocate people to the space that they occupy in Your Circle of Influence; you can also begin to consider whether they are a largely Positive or a largely Negative Influence.

Is there anyone or any activity that you feel affects your persistent weight problem in a Positive or a Negative way?

> What you need to understand about Influencing Factors is that you don't need to be spending all your time with them; for them to be having a big impact on you.
>
> Also the ones who are having the Biggest Impact on you; do not have to be the closest to you.

So what do I want you to take away from this chapter?

We all have a Circle of Influence which spreads out from ourselves.

Within that Circle of Influence we have Influencing Factors.

These Influencing Factors can be people, their behaviour, their attitudes, their opinions, the way that they Do things and the Things that they want.

We can often be Influenced in a Positive or Negative way without realising that we are being so influenced.

We all have relationships which are Positive and relationships which are Negative.

Very few relationships are purely wholly Positive (Beneficial) or wholly Negative (Detrimental). Most relationships are made up of both of these.

However; most relationships will have an overall pattern to them which is such that; when we look at them honestly, will put them into the Positive or Negative Relationship categories.

As we become more aware of our Circle of Influence and our Influencing Factors, we can begin to Evaluate them and Move them in Directions which are More Beneficial for us.

CHAPTER 22

Problems With Different Time Frames

There are lots of human related problems. The variations and variety of them is staggering.

So it should come as no surprise that persistent Weight Problems also have lots of variations and varieties.

When we look at the Spectrum of Weight Problems there are weight problems which we can easily place and say; Yes that goes there on the Spectrum.

Then there are those weight problems which are Confusing and difficult to place.

These confusing problems don't seem to fit the obvious patterns and structures but seem to have Components of those patterns and structures.

It would seem as if these problems only occur in certain situations; at certain times or when certain Human Dynamics are involved.

This can be difficult for many people to deal with as we live in a society where we have become used to Labelling Conditions and Behaviours.

These problems however; seem to defy easy labelling. So let's call these:

Episodic and Irregular Problems.

What can be confusing about Episodic and Irregular Problems is that they may occur for a short period of time every few months or even every few years.

The Impact of the problem can be very Intense and High; but for a short period of time.

Episodic Problems can also seem to "Just Appear" with no apparent justification.

Episodic Problems can also be Covered Up quite easily but they can build up a history that becomes "The Elephant in the Room".

It becomes something that people are aware of; but No-One is able to deal with the Problem effectively and it is allowed to Just Exist.

What can happen with this dynamic is that the size of the Elephant can then begin to vary. Sometimes it gets bigger and other times it gets smaller.

Another thing that can happen is that this type of problem can continue for many years and even decades without being properly addressed.

When this happens it can become "Normalised" as being A Part of the Lifestyle of the person and of the family as well.

It can then move to a point where it is considered to be a Normal Part of the Person and Who They Are.

We can then move to the position of:

It's just something I have to live with!

So how do we begin to understand these problems so that we can begin to work with them?

Let's keep it simple!

Does the problem have a food component?

Is someone over eating, under eating or switching their diet?

What's the frequency?

What's the impact on their lifestyle?

And we can go on asking simple questions and building a picture of the problem and the impact of the problem.

In my experience there is often an element of "Game Playing" with these problems.

When I use the term Game Playing what I am saying is that events, circumstances, relationships and people may be being controlled, manipulated or managed by others.

So this is something that we need to be aware of.

Game Playing also occurs with all the other weight related problems, all along the Spectrum of Weight Problems; so this is nothing new or unusual.

Often a good place to begin understanding and working with these problems is to start with the

Impact on the person's Lifestyle and the Lifestyle of others.

Other techniques and tools can then help us to understand the problem in depth.

What can make these problems difficult is that Episodic Problems may occur prior to, at the time of, or subsequent to annual events or anniversaries of events.

Also there can be a Disconnection in the persons mind between the Problem and the Casual Factors which leads to the Materialisation of the Problem itself.

This type of problem is one that the Dieters Scale and the Human Dynamics Matrix helps us to understand, manage and resolve.

We haven't looked at the Human Dynamics Matrix© yet but the Dieters Scale© is giving you an introduction to it.

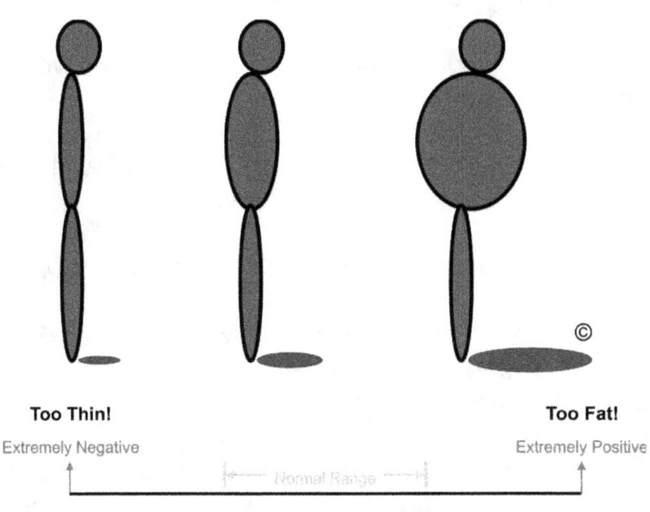

The Spectrum of Weight Problems

So what do I want you to take away from this chapter?

Episodic problems can leave the people who have them, feeling as if they are isolated.

In reality Episodic problems are just problems with an Episodic Structure.

Episodic Structures can be understood and worked with; just like any other problem can be.

Periodic Problems will fit into the Dieters Scale©.

And they will fit into the Human Dynamics Matrix© which allows us to look at them in more detail and in greater depth.

Periodic Problems can have all the same difficulties that any Amber Zone or Red Zone problem would have.

What is extremely unlikely is that the Episodic Problem can be deal with without dealing with other directly and indirectly related Human Dynamics.

If you are suffering from an Episodic Problem there are people out there who can help.

My advice would be to avoid the Quick Fixes which you will no doubt be offered.

CHAPTER 23

Body Dysmorphia And Social And General Dysmorphia

Distorted and Inaccurate perceptions are normal in everyday life.

When we are the person who is experiencing these distorted and inaccurate perceptions; they can be as real to us as any solid brick wall.

And when we run into them, they can have the same Effect and Affect as running into a solid brick wall would have.

They can Affect us Emotionally. Causing problems with different aspects of how we perceive ourselves in different situations. And how we perceive ourselves as worthy and credible people; and reflect upon how we perceive our place and position in the world.

They can Effect us in the Actions that we take and the behaviours that we employ with ourselves and with others.

Like so many other human conditions Dysmorphia is something that has a number of different Components.

To my mind; Dysmorphia is a structured view of certain things that can be informed by particular insecurities, anxieties, stresses, beliefs, facts and circumstances.

The mixture of the components which create the structure of the Dysmorphia can determine the Form that it takes.

The Form is simply how we would choose to label what is being experienced by the person.

With some people it is labelled and called Body Dysmorphia.

Body Dysmorphia is when, either in reality or in their view of things, someone believes that parts of their body are in some way not normal.

This real or perceived abnormality can also go with an increased sensitivity and awareness to their view of their physical form and how others may perceive them.

This can then lead on to further problems in their attempts to manage and address their concerns.

Dysmorphia only really becomes a problem when it escalates and moves to another level. To help you understand this I am going to use a comparative example.

A comparative example would be:

> Someone with a small weight problem would be in the Green Zone on The Dieters Scale©. This would be a Low level problem.
>
> And someone with a large weight problem would be in the Red Zone on The Dieters Scale©. This would be a Higher level problem.

So both have a weight problem but of different degrees.

> The person with the Green Zone weight problem would have less Consequences from their weight problem and would normally have fewer Associated Problems. They also have less weight to lose.
>
> The person with the Red Zone weight problem would have more Consequences from their weight problem and would normally have More Associated Problems. They, comparatively, have more weight to lose.

So we are seeing and measuring the difference between the two Zones by The Dieters Scale and the Impact on the person from the Consequences of the persistent weight problem.

Problems occur when the person with the Green Zone problems believes themselves to be someone living in the Red Zone and tries to lose too much weight.

Body Dysmorphia can form part of a Weight Problem that someone experiences. When this occurs it is simply a Component of the overall problem that need to be worked with.

Problems with Dysmorphia related to weight would normally be associated with the Too Thin end of The Spectrum of Weight Problems (Someone underweight) but I think that it actually spans the whole Spectrum.

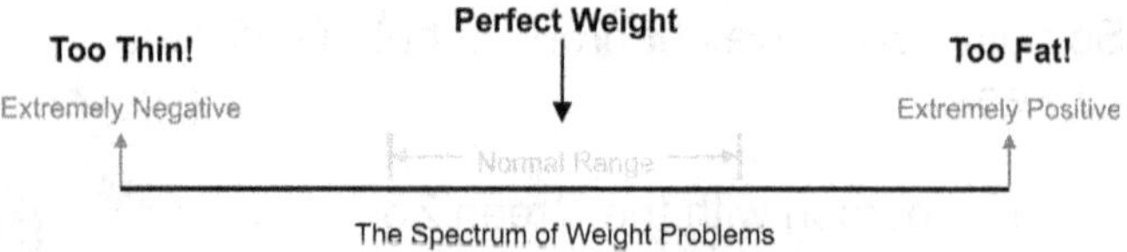

My view is that we can apply a scale to Dysmorphia and use this to help us understand and work with it; in the same way that we would do so with a weight problem.

The more that I look at people and the Human Condition, the more that I am sure that Dysmorphia permeates what we do and influences us more than we realise.

How much better would we be at understanding and dealing with situations; if we understood that it is our Perception of the Reality of those situations, and our Perception the role of ourselves in those situations that may need some work?

> In a sense; Dysmorphia means that we miss-frame, miss-understand, miss-perceive and miss-construct our Internal picture of the world in which we participate.

Not only does our picture become distorted; but the way that we interact with the world and the impact of our involvement in the world can also be affected.

> We do say that Reality is whatever you believe it to be. And sometimes that belief is accurate and at other times it is based on faulty and misleading information.

For my own view of Dysmorphia, I think that it probably extends into all areas of human activity.

For example:

Someone finds themselves in a situation where they are feeling vulnerable, lacking in confidence, experiencing low self-esteem and having a mental image of themselves that corresponds with the low self-esteem, low confidence and feelings of vulnerability that they are experiencing.

> Are they seeing a mental image of themselves doing something wrong and being embarrassed by the result?
>
> Are they sensitive to a blemish on their skin that they are sure that everyone must surely see?
>
> Are they in a situation where their lack of formal education or qualifications makes them sensitive and over aware of their surroundings and the people they are going to meet?

In a one-off situation we may accept nerves as an answer and move on with life.

But what happens when it isn't a one-off and it happens more often?

When do we Cross the Threshold from an Acceptable Problem to an Unacceptable Problem?

Does it make it easier to understand and work with certain types of problems; if we say that the person is experiencing a form of Dysmorphia that is normal?

In my example above where we have the components of low self-esteem, low confidence and feelings of vulnerability.

Were we to attempt to deal with each of these individually; would we actually deal with the problem?

Reality is Subjective. Many of the problems that we experience as people occur from that Subjective experiencing of Reality.

What we benefit from as people is learning that all of this is Normal and that we can influence, change and improve how we perceive the world and our place in it.

However; it will not necessarily be an easy thing to do!

So what do I want you to take away from this chapter?

> As a result of all the different Components of a problem coming together; we have problems that can take on a life and character of their own.
>
> If we can better understand the points of Confluence (where things come together), then we can modify them to achieve more beneficial outcomes.

Dysmorphia is something that we are still trying to understand.

Like all problems it has its own unique structures that move it one way or another way.

I am reminded of that saying:

> The Whole is greater than the Sum of its Parts.

Problems can be just like that. They produce something extra as a result of different Components coming together.

And like any problem; when we begin to work with the Structure and the Components which make up that structure: We can then begin to Change the Structure and Change what the structure Produces.

It just takes time, effort and the Correct Application Of Actions to do so!

CHAPTER 24

Going Through: “The Shredder!”

Those of you who have a problem that falls into the Green Zone may not understand this.

Those of you who have a problem that falls into the Amber and Red Zones should have an idea of what I am talking about; and many of you will know it well.

So what is it?

When you deal with and want to change certain types of problems, you simply cannot avoid Discomfort.

By managing the different processes, you can reduce the levels of discomfort and take many of the edges off of it, but you cannot eliminate all of the discomfort.

To avoid the discomfort many people will do things like; seek medication, begin drinking more or have an increased impulse to eat and consume certain foods.

This can be a Danger Period because this is a time where one type of undesirable behaviour can be replaced by another type of undesirable behaviour.

In the drugs and alcohol field this is a time where people can: Switch Addictions.

When someone Switches Addictions it does not have to be from one substance to another. It can be that they use a behaviour to replace a substance.

For example someone may use Exercise and throw themselves into it.

Other people may choose to Cook, become more Religious, want more Intimacy and Sex, begin Cleaning more and so on.

What I have seen is that this type of behaviour can appear to be doing the job; but because of how it is being used and what it is being expected to do:

> It cannot sustain itself. And it crashes and the person is back where they began or perhaps further back and in more of a mess.

The reality is that none of us can avoid the discomfort of change but we have the ability to manage it and understand what is happening while it occurs.

Change is often a difficult process to experience; even if it is Change which is wanted and desired.

A simple reason for this is:

> That you are going to change your Normal Unwanted behaviour to a New Normal Wanted Behaviour.
>
> To achieve this you are going to move from one place to another.

So if you prepare for and accept that there are going to be times when you will have to:

Go through The Shredder!

Then when you do so it becomes less difficult.

Why do I call it The Shredder?

I call it this simply because this is what it can feel like at times.

> The good news is that if you follow the right processes for dealing with the problem; that you can get through The Shredder and complete the transitions in a better way.
>
> There also tend to be less Repeats of behaviour due to failure; which means that you don't have to keep going through it.

What you also need to understand is this:

You may hit The Shredder a number of different times and in different ways as you encounter and deal with the different aspects and components of your individual persistent weight problem.

So what do I want you to take away from this chapter?

Depending on where you are starting from and the degree of your problems; sooner or later, most of us hit The Shedder!

A good way to think of it is like Turbulence experienced by an airplane as it flies in the air.

Turbulence can make the journey unpleasant and scary but most people land safely and in one piece; if they stay in their seats and complete their journey.

Those who jump out of the planes when it gets unpleasant may avoid being bumped about; but now what?

CHAPTER 25

Are You A Secret Eater, Boozer, In Denial…

Whenever we deal with difficult problems, we always have to be aware of certain difficult realities that exist.

Many of these difficult realities relate to behaviours that we have developed, fallen into, join in with or are forced into adopting.

For many people, using these behaviours is what gets them through. It helps them to survive another day.

When someone is looking at changing, improving and developing their lives in a better way; we reach a point where these difficult behaviours can begin to undermine the work being done to achieve that new life.

In reality: We all reach a point where we need to deal with the difficult behaviours that may be being kept secret or hidden.

Usually this is not as difficult as people think it is going to be.

Those difficult behaviours I am talking about include:

- Lies.

- Deceptions.
- Denial.
- No Cognitive Awareness.
- Fear of Engaging with Difficult Issues.
- Living On Auto-Pilot.
- Not being allowed to be Who or What you really are.

The reality in life is that no-one is perfect.

Other people may do things better than you, you may do things better than other people, and so on.

From your perspective you may think that other people are perfect and that you should be; or that you are so imperfect that you will never be any good.

The reality may be that you have thoughts like this but the truth is that absolutely no-one on this planet; either now, in the past or in the future; will be perfect in every way and behave perfectly all the time.

It's an Impossible Standard of Behaviour.

To hold yourself to an Impossible Standard of Behaviour is a sure way to make sure that your fail.

I have a saying that I use for myself. It is:

> Excellence when required; Good enough when appropriate!

In this world the reality is that we are dealing with Imperfect People. And Imperfect People make mistakes and do things that are Not Perfect.

Another reality is that we all hide things and we all have secrets.

This is normal.

The reality is:

> Every day you get the Opportunity to write another chapter in Your Life Profile and develop a new style future without the secret behaviour.
>
> And you get the Opportunity to stop having to live in the old chapters of Your Life Profile.

Another reality of Life is that:

> Sometimes the Right Thing is not the Easy Thing to do.

I know that from my own life experiences.

> But we all reach a point where we find that we have chosen to make a stand and we then make choices which can be life changing.

It simply becomes a choice of what is Right for You.

When I work with these issues in a Life Improvement Programme I take the following approach:

> I am going to address these difficult realities in a Non-Judgemental and Non-Blaming way; and treat them as just being the Realities that certain people will experience and that they will be living with.

Whatever behaviour someone has, if it is a problem for them and/or the people that they live with; then normally something can be done to help improve, resolve or better manage the behaviour.

Just remember that it is not always going to be easy.

There are a myriad of ways that people can use problematic and difficult behaviours. What I am interested in here are ones that will fall within the scope of this book.

This would be the following type of behaviours.

For example; are you:

A Boozer.
Secret Eater.
In Denial.
Automatic grazer of Food and Drinks.
Binge eater.
Someone who Purges.
Someone who Fast.
Someone who Self-harms.

These are just examples and there are many more of these types of behaviour out there.

So what do I want you to take away from this chapter?

If you have a persistent weight problem then it is, in my experience, normal to have other problems and issues as well.

You may have already tried to deal with your weight problem and the other issues that cause you difficulties. And you may have had some temporary success.

With complex problems you reach a point where you cannot continue to make choices about dealing only with one part of the problem.

This is because the Nature of the problem has changed to a point where this is no longer possible to do.

What you need to avoid doing; is to continually try to use the same old solution that keeps on failing.

So you need to think in terms of a new type of solution.

This is why I developed the Life Improvement Programmes; to provide a way of successfully dealing with complex problems.

CHAPTER 26

An Introduction To The Human Dynamics Matrix©

As you have read through this book, you will have become familiar with The Dieters Scale©.

The Dieters Scale© allows us to begin to look at and understand the structure of a persistent weight problem.

It also allows us to begin seeing the detail of the problem and it helps us to look at the different Components of the problem.

And as we do this, we begin to get an idea of what we need to do to resolve, improve and manage this problem in a different way.

For lots of people this will be a massive leap forwards and it may help them deal with their problem in another way. Which is great!

For me however; this was not enough!

The Dieters Scale© can be very useful and very helpful. But it doesn't actually give me the real information and detail that I really need to deal with Amber Zone and Red Zone problems.

It also doesn't give me the real information that I need to help someone in the Green Zone from moving into the Amber or Red Zones.

To do this; I needed an innovative, reliable, high quality, more refined, accurate and robust way of understanding the structure and nature of problems in the different Zones.

I wanted to find a way that would help me see the structure of these problems and then lead on to the structure of the solutions.

I also wanted to be able to create an accurate record of the process and create a process with Predictability!

This was not available and so I had to create it.

What I was actually looking for was a New Methodology for working with Psycho-somatic problems.

And it took a number of innovative steps for me to create what I was after.

> My book: An Introduction To The Human Dynamics Matrix; goes into more details about this and it explains more about The Human Dynamics Matrix. This book is on limited release.

You see; apart from weight problems, we have many other problems which have very high failure rates, when solutions are applied to them.

What is common in all of these different types of problems is the people and the dynamics which they cause and bring with them to the problem.

So I was looking for a solution that could be applied to these different complicated Human problems; and not just persistent weight problems.

> I realised that if I thought about problems in a different way, that I could begin to work with them in a different way.

And over a period of time I created The Human Dynamics Matrix and the methodology that goes with it to enable me to work with Psycho-somatic problems.

So what is different about this approach?

I am going to keep this simple and just use a few graphics to help you understand.

With The Dieters Scale we used 3 colours: Red, Amber and Green to illustrate that things are different from one Zone to another Zone.

We could use other colours and we could use more colour but for general purposes 3 colours and 3 Zones works well.

So far, we have asked the 6 questions we had at the beginning of this book and we put the answers into columns to create a graph.

This helps us outline the problem at a basic level but there is more actually going on which we need to see and understand.

When you really begin working with the Nature of problems, you find that problems have Shapes.

They have Shapes because problems go in different directions.

- A Positive Direction.
- A Negative Direction.
- Moving Forwards.
- Moving Backwards.

Problems also occupy certain spaces and have supporting structures.

And they also have a few other things as well.

So to work with a persistent weight problem effectively, we need to understand the nature of the weight problem. And get to the structure that supports what it is doing.

> And all of these parts may be moving independently and in different directions.

So you see that this can quickly get complicated.

But we can simplify it all by applying the right Methodology and tools.

A Methodology is simply the consistent application of a process; which can be measured, recorded and repeated.

So if we go back to The Zones of The Dieters Scale©.

And we look at the Range over which problems spread.

The circle shows the reality; that problems can spread in all directions from the centre outwards.

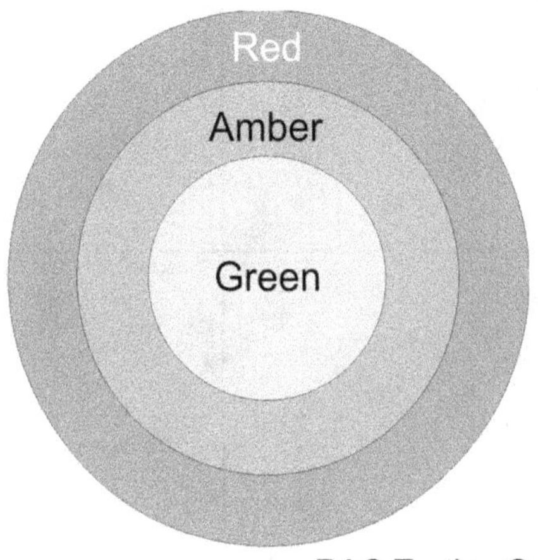

RAG Testing ©

So you can see that when we use The Dieters Scale, we can see the Zone circle that something may belong in.

But we can't see whereabouts it is in the Zone circle and what is the Relevance of it being there?

To understand this we have to create a Structure that can make sense of this.

The structure shown below is what enables us make sense of this and to get more helpful and useful information.

This graphic shows the Graph structure for the Human Dynamics Matrix© that I created.

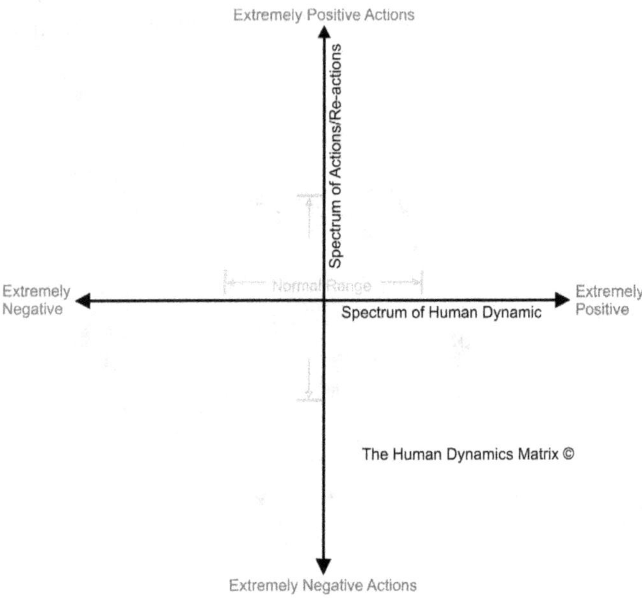

I am not going to go into much detail here but the reality is that this structure, when it is properly used, can give us a lot of insight and depth of understanding.

In the next graphic I am going to bring The Dieters Zones and the above graphic together.

And when we bring these together we get we get something which resembles: “A Target”.

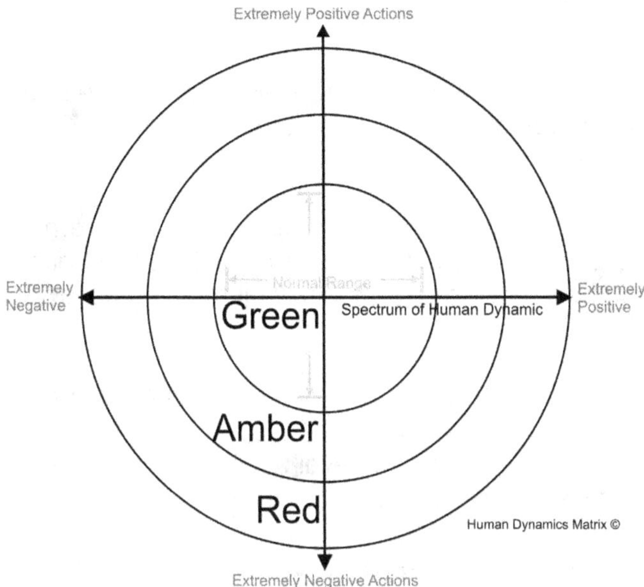

This structure then enable me to place all the activities of the persistent weight problem and the associated activities and problems that go with it; on the graph.

This then enables me to build up a map of the different components of the problem; and we can see how the different components Effect and Affect both the person and their problem.

The Human Dynamics Matrix let's me map out each component, for example Self-Esteem. And it allows me to map out the entire Weight Problem and its components:

> The Human Dynamics Matrix also shows me the Nature of the problem and the Nature of the actions that the person has been taking.

The Human Dynamics Matrix also lets me see and understand the Long Term Tendencies of someone's activities.

Understanding whether someone has a long term Tendency towards Positive or Negative behaviour and how that directly effects what they are doing is a very important thing.

Being able to extend this and work with a weight problem and all the associated problems and issues; lets me get to a level of detail which is very useful and productive.

> Once we can see all this, then we can work out exactly what needs to be changed and how it needs to be changed.

So I am using the Human Dynamics Matrix Methodology© to achieve a understanding of a single person's problem structure and the structure of the solution that they personally need to resolve, improve or manage their problem.

And I am using the Methodology to achieve a better understanding of the different stages of Weight Problems on the Spectrum of Weight Problems. I.e. This process helps to create a profile for the different parts of the Weight Spectrum.

This enables me to then build up this information into a useful resource.

So what do I want you to take away from this chapter?

The Dieters Scale helps us to understand someone's weight problem using Zones.

However; for many weight problems we need to understand the problem at a different level and with more detail than Zones alone can provide.

The Human Dynamics Matrix lets us get to that different level and those details.

The Human Dynamics Matrix lets us provide an Individually Tailored Solution to someone with a persistent weight problem.

We can go further than conventional diet and weight control programmes because we can work with all the different components of a weight problem and not just the obvious ones.

The Human Dynamics Matrix© also facilitates Experiential Learning; and it helps with achieving Insights into problems and their management.

CHAPTER 27

Putting It All Together

So how do you put all this information and new thinking together?

If there is a message that I have been trying to get across in this book, it is that things happen a bit more slowly than people want and often in a different way than they think they do.

If I was in your place what would I do?

First I would read through the whole of this book without skipping bits. And I would allow thinking time while I read it.

Then if I thought I needed to: I would read it again.

I would keep the book available so that I could refer to relevant chapters.

I would understand The Dieters Scale© and I would answer the simple questions.

I would try to see where I think my persistent weight problem and the other problems are within the different Zones of The Dieters Scale©.

Before I did anything I would make sure that I understood whether I thought my weight problem was a Green Zone, Amber Zone or Red Zone problem.

I would expect that as I went from the Green Zone to the Amber and Red Zone; that my problem is going to get more difficult, more complex and is going to take more time to deal with.

I would accept that I don't have a weight problem that exist in isolation to other things. I would ask:

> What Components does my persistent weight problem have and where do I think these are on The Dieters Scale?

I would then look at the options that I am considering using to deal with my problem.

- Am I considering another diet?
- What pressure am I putting myself under?
- How long am I allowing myself to deal with this problem?
- What am I going to be relying upon?
- Do I need to do something different?
- Why am I doing this now?

Then I would look at "When" I was going to do this.

I would be asking the questions: Is there something else which is driving this decision?

I would also be looking at how I am going to deal with the various issues which may have been raised throughout this book.

I would also accept that I might begin this and that I might follow my usual path and stop when things get difficult.

If I did that, then I would read the section about Imperfect People again.

At some point I would have to accept that:

> If I keep doing the same sort of thing and I keep getting the same sort of result; then at some point I will need to do something quite different in order to achieve something different.

And this may be what has brought you to this book:

> You are Looking for something else that you can do to sort this weight problem out.

Whatever you do just remember this simple truth:

> If you participate in the Solution to your problem in the right ways; then you can resolve, improve or manage your weight problem in a better way.

So what do I want you to take away from this chapter?

- Be realistic.
- Don't be over optimistic.
- Virtually all weight related problems can be dealt with.

CHAPTER 28

Choose Who, What And How You Want To Be; From Now On!

One of the great things about a persistent weight problem is:

> That at some point: You get to make choices about Your life and Your place in the World.

You will have done this already; perhaps several times.

It will have happened as the problem developed and you may not have been aware of the significance of your choices at the time.

Making these choices doesn't happen all at once; it happens gradually as you move from one stage of the problem to another stage.

You may not have been aware that you were making these choices but you were actively making them.

As you made these choices you would have been unaware of the long term consequences of those choices. This is because these things tend to happen slowly.

Because these things happen slowly we don't have the Contrasting Picture between our lives now and what they will become in the future.

If we had that Contrasting Picture, then we would probably make different and better decisions.

When we sit down and begin to think about the future and how we want our lives to change; we are, in effect, creating that Contrasting Picture.

And we are seeing ourselves in that Picture and making decisions about it. For example:

> Now my life is like this!
> In the future I want my life to be more like that.

In the early stage of changing, improving and better managing a life, it is easier.

We can make rapid and fairly easy changes if things are in a mess.

It is when we move beyond the early stage and we move into the next and following stages that Structure, Objectives, Motivation and Purpose become very Important.

It is the second and following stages that most people struggle with.

For example:

> It is fairly easy to begin a new diet and exercise programme. You can achieve quick results and feel great about it.

After a short while these rapid results begin to fade and then you approach a new stage in the process.

This is when many people begin to fail.

What many of the Self-help and Motivational Guru's fail to tell people is; that Change, Improvement and Getting a better life; can be very, very difficult at times.

In fact; Difficult is the reality of this for most people.

Unbelievably Difficult is the reality for a lot of people.

And Impossibly Difficult is the reality for others.

But once again all of these can be Managed.

Let's go back to The Dieters Scale©.

Put Difficult into the Green Zone. It's normal.

Put Unbelievably Difficult into the Amber Zone.

Put Impossibly Difficult into the Red Zone.

Now it's a bit less scary!

You see what people make a mistake with is that they look at their lives and they see it as all being at the same level.

But lives are not One Dimensional they are Multi-Dimensional.

You will live certain parts of your life in the Green Zone. Other parts of your life will be lived in the Amber and Red Zones.

You simply cannot treat each of these as being the same!

If you do:

Then your chances of Failing Increases!

So when you do make those choices about Who, How and What you want to be from now on, and in the future:

> Make sure that you understand the Contrast between where you are Now and where you want to Be in the Future.
>
> Don't be afraid to admit that certain things that you need or want to do are bigger, scarier and more difficult than others. It's normal for that to be the case.
>
> Look at the different aspects of your life and see what belongs in the Green Zone, what belongs in the Amber Zone and what belongs in the Red Zone.
>
> Accept that these may need to be deal with and managed in different ways.

The Key Decision that every person will make at different stages of their lives, whether they realise it or not is:

> Am I going to be Pro-Active and really go for this properly; or not?

So what do I want you to take away from this chapter?

You have the opportunity to choose Who, How and What you want To Be from now on.

You really, really do have that opportunity.

But no-one is going to achieve this for you. You have to achieve it yourself.

You need to think that you are on your life journey and that you are going to determine the Direction, Purpose and Quality of that journey from now onwards.

If you fail to make those decisions and to take the necessary actions to make them into a reality; then you will be left with what other people and society lets you have.

CHAPTER 29

The Real Timeline For Becoming The Person You Want To Be

Let's have a look at what I think is likely to be the Real Timeline for:

Becoming The Person You Really Want To Be.

To be realistic with this we need to qualify a few things.

Those who fall into the Green Zone on The Dieters Scale© should have a less complex, less embedded and less difficult problem mix; than someone who falls into the Amber Zone and the Red Zone.

What I am talking about here is not only the Weight Problem that the person has; but also all the other directly and indirectly affected areas of life which contribute towards the development and maintenance of the Persistent Weight Problem.

And which are also Effected and Affected by the Persistent Weight Problem.

So I am looking at the Whole Problem and not just the Weight Part.

I am looking at what we need to do to deal with the persistent weight problem and what we need to do so as not to come back to this place again.

At what point would someone expect to have Turned The Corner and Really be taking their Life in a Different, Sustainable Direction?

We are looking at being truthful here and not giving people false expectations. So I will tell you what I really think and what my experience shows me.

To answer the question I am also going to use The Dieters Scale©.

We should now have established that life is like a Jigsaw with different pieces which fit together.

Those different pieces can have different shapes, sizes and colours.

To make sense of this we have used Green, Amber and Red Zones.

So when we look at the Jigsaw of our own lives and we look at the different shapes, sizes and colours of the different issues, problems, changes and challenges that we need to deal with; we will find that we have a colour map.

That map may be more Green, more Amber or more Red than someone else's.

As an indicator; I would say that if our Map is genuinely all Green that it can be dealt with in 1-year with the Correct Application of Actions.

As an indicator; I would say that if our Map has bits that are Amber that it can be dealt with in 1- 2 years or less with the Correct Application of Actions.

As an indicator; I would say that if our Map has bits that are Red that it can be dealt with in 1-3 years or less with the Correct Application of Actions.

Now all of this is just a guide but why not ask yourself if it really seems realistic to you; that all of your problems are going to be dealt with simply, easily and quickly?

If they could; then you would simply, quickly and easily have dealt with them.

The timelines also begin from when you actually begin to properly begin to deal with these things.

> Some problems may defy these guidelines and that is why these are only guidelines.
>
> Some problems may take years to deal with.
>
> Other problems may not be able to be dealt with and can only be better managed.
>
> Each case is different and each case has different dynamics attached to it.

When we get to this level of successfully dealing with long term problems; you may well need help.

This is because there is simply “a lot of things going on” and many of those things are going to be outside of your current awareness and your current ability to comprehend. This is Normal.

So what do I want you to take away from this chapter?

If you decide to use The Dieters Scale© to grade the different problems, issues and challenges that you have; then be realistic.

Green Zone level problems are the simplest and easiest to deal with.

As you Unpack and begin to deal with a problem; you may find that the Nature of the problem actually changes; and that it is not actually a Green Zone problem but an Amber or Red Zone problem.

You could also find that one problem is sitting inside of another problem.

Amber and Red Zone problems are more complicated, more difficult and more complex to deal with and they usually take longer.

With many problems an Annual Cycle is required so as to deal with things like Anniversaries of Events.

Things like Christmas, holidays and birthdays can trigger problem dynamics that are not there the whole year through.

More complicated problems may require more than one Annual Cycle.

CHAPTER 30

Life Improvement Programmes

With many problems we try the quickest, simplest and easiest solutions first.

And for many problems these quick, simple and easy solutions work just fine.

So why should Life Problems be any different.

Well the reality is that for many Life Problems there are quick, simple and easy solutions that can be successfully applied.

The real problems begin when we reach the stage where we run out of quick, simple and easy solutions to apply.

Or: When the nature of the problem is such that quick, simple and easy solutions are no longer appropriate.

What do we do when we reach this stage?

For myself; as an innovator, developer and provider of solutions; I found that many of the solutions being offered to different problems were badly structured, inadequate, over sold and often unable to do the job.

I saw that people with Red Zone problems were being sold Green Zone solutions.

This doesn't only happen with weight problems, it happens all through society.

- Businesses get sold and buy the wrong solutions.
- Governments get sold and buy the wrong solutions.
- People get sold and buy the wrong solutions.

It happens to be a Normal thing. However; just because it's normal, it doesn't make it right.

Over the last 25-years I have been developing Lifestyle Management Solutions.

I began developing these because I could see that there were certain types of problems that required more than a conventional solution could provide.

I have to say that doing this has been something of an uphill struggle quite a lot of the time.

Have you ever heard the saying:

> Just because something is good for someone; it doesn't mean that they will want it.

And this is true for all sorts of solutions to problems.

Let me give you an example:

> If you have someone shouting loudly and offering people with weight problems a simple, quick, painless solution; then they will have a

long queue of people lining up to buy it from them.

If you offer people a very effective long term solution that is innovative, high quality and reliable; but it is not quick, easy and simple:

Then you will have very few people queuing up to buy it.

This is simple human nature at work.

If I offer you something which taste sweet and I tell you it will cure your problem; you will take this over someone else offering you something which taste sour to cure the same problem.

And this is how it is with Lifestyle Management Solutions.

They are great solutions but because they are dealing with difficult issues they are not always sweet. They simply can't be!

To get people using Lifestyle Management Solutions we have to go through a process of Education.

We have to help people see the benefits of solutions which do more than conventional solutions; but which can also be sour at times.

Think of Life Improvement Programmes as being a evolution out of Lifestyle Management Solutions.

They have been created to work with the complex mix that can occur with problems across the Spectrum of Weight Problems.

They are designed to work with The Dieters Scale and the complicated mixture of Green, Amber and Red Zone problems that people actually have.

With a Life Improvement Programme we are recognising and accepting that the problem mix we are looking at and working with; involves the person at a fundamental level.

This is because the person is the key part in the process and it is their Life that is important.

Working in this way involves working with the Management, Development and Structure of their life.

In everything we do, we are focused on the long term goal of the Life Improvement Programme.

Whether our final goal is freedom from dieting or another aspect of life or personal achievement.

For example:

Where it is a Life Improvement Programme focused on Weight. We will have successfully dealing with that, as our long term focus but not our exclusive focus. We will address other issues as well.

So what do I want you to take away from this chapter?

Problems are not all sweetness, sunshine and laughter.

So why would you expect the solution to be all sweetness, sunshine and laughter?

Life Improvement Programmes which are properly structured and delivered can make significant differences to Life problems that many people have.

If you are going to undertake a Life Improvement Programme you need to understand the commitment involved and NOT be looking for quick, simple, easy results.

Extraordinary results can be delivered but it is through a sweet and sour process that takes time.

CHAPTER 31

Lifestyle, Wealth, Health And Well-Being!

For a large part of my life I have been looking at and working with the structures that are required for achieving more successful lives.

I have developed an eye for the structures of success; and I have been developing structures that are required for being successful with resolving, improving and managing problems.

Over that time; I have found that there are many people who will tell you that they have the secrets to success of various types.

They can provide you with 100 easy ways to be successful with making money, persuading people to do things, losing weight, being happier, etc.

Then there are the people who will tell you that they can make you; A Winner!

They will tell you that being A Winner is what being successful in life is all about.

In my opinion; the reality is actually simpler and more achievable.

> It's not about being A Winner.
> It's not about finding a 100 easy ways to...

In reality:

> Successful, Happy lives are about Balance.
>
> A balanced life is generally a happier life than one which is out of balance.

Over the years I have realised that we can break life down into four simple Areas which connect together. These are:

> Lifestyle, Wealth, Health and Well-Being.

If we can get these different areas of our lives to balance with what we want to achieve in life; then we tend to be successful.

If we neglect any of these four areas, then our lives go out of balance and we suffer the consequences of this.

> I can safely say that when people have problems, one or more of these areas is going to be out of balance.

So if you have a weight problem then one of more of these areas in your life is going to be out of balance.

So let's take a simple look at these four areas.

Lifestyle

Lifestyle is made up from the structures of our lives on a day-by-day basis.

It's the coming together of the little insignificant parts of our lives and the larger more significant parts of our lives.

When these combine, they help to define us as people and the type of Lifestyle that we have.

It includes the Routines and Habits of our daily living.

Lifestyle includes such things as; shopping for groceries, cleaning the house, looking after the children, looking after our partner, our parents, etc.

All the things which we would normally take for granted in our lives; such as preparing food, watching TV, speaking to people on the phone are part of our Lifestyle.

It also includes things like hobbies, sports and our social lives.

The habits we have around work are also part of our lifestyle. Including getting out of bed in the morning, going to work and what we do after work.

Lifestyle includes the relationships that we have at home, at work and in the general communities which we inhabit.

It would also include On-Line relationships and communities that we use.

So Lifestyle covers a large part of our life and if there are things in our Lifestyles which are wrong; then they can affect this area and other areas.

If you were to think about your Lifestyle and then you were to apply The Dieters Scale to the different areas of your Lifestyle:

> Which parts of your Lifestyle would be in the Green, Amber or Red Zones?

Wealth

In all of our lives we have to pay some attention to wealth. Either in getting it, spending it or both of these.

This is simply because we all need money to live and we all have bills to pay.

Wealth covers:

> Our Income.
> Savings.
> Investments.
> Inheritance.
> Other people's finances which effects us.
> Our work and the means by which we earn money.
> Taxes.
>
> It also covers:
>
> Our expenditure.
> Our Liabilities.

Financial Commitments.
Unexpected Expenditure.

As we move through our life our wealth requirements change and we all eventually give up working.

In most households someone will have a job or be living with someone who has a job.

In the current economic climate many people are relying on assistance from other people or State organisations.

Many people are defined by the Possessions that they have and that they enjoy.

If those Possessions are removed or lost; what then?

Many people are defined by what they do to make a living. Their Occupational Status defines who they are and their Occupational Status links to their ability to create wealth.

Where this is the case; what happens when someone loses their job or cannot work anymore?

When people manage their wealth poorly, they tend to suffer at some point. Sometimes poor management leads to bankruptcy and other times it leads to permanent financial stress.

Virtually everyone is capable of paying sufficient attention to their finances; and they are capable of learning how to manage them well.

For anyone who has had the experience of not having money that they need. Then we know that:

> The quality of our lives can be affected by not having enough money.

And another truth is:

> Sometimes; someone's Lifestyle demands financing which outpaces the ability of their wealth creation.

Another thing about wealth is:

> Successful people may become wealthy.
>
> However; being wealthy doesn't make you a successful person.

I have come to realise that few people will really become fabulously wealthy. And that although many people would like the advantages of being wealthy, this is not really what they want.

Most people that I talk to about being wealthy actually just want to be better off than they are now and not have to worry about money.

If you were to think about your Wealth and then you were to apply The Dieters Scale© to the different areas of your Wealth:

> Which parts of your Wealth would be in the Green, Amber or Red Zones?

Health

Under Health we would include:

> Physical Health.
> Mental Health.
> Emotional Health.
> Psychological Health.

We know that health concerns can drive us to take action through fear. Health concerns may well have made you read this book.

Good health does not exist in isolation to our Lifestyles or our Wealth. Our lifestyles and our Wealth contribute towards our health and helps to shape it over the medium to long term.

Things like a weight problem can cause us long term physical health problems.

> Weight problems and the associated physiological problems are obviously physical in their nature.
>
> But health problems are not exclusively physical.

I personally believe that we should do what we can to maintain our health and to address any health concerns that we have.

Good health is something that most of us tend to take for granted. It is only when we are not well that we have the contrast between Good Health and Poor Health.

Dealing with a weight problem is something that you have a choice over doing; the question is:

Will you take it seriously this time?

Persistent weight problems can affect all the areas shown at the beginning of this section.

This means that they can affect our Mental, Emotional, Psychological and Physical Health.

Because many health problems occur over time; we may not appreciate that we are helping to create a long term health problem through our current behaviour.

Very often it is only in the future that we will make these connections.

At that time we will be able to see that what we have done in the past has contributed to or caused the thing which is now dragging down our lives.

> A simple long term health problem can cause our quality of life to reduce and it can make us miserable. So if we can avoid this; why not?

If you were to think about your Health and then you were to apply The Dieters Scale© to the different areas of your Health:

> Which parts of your Health would be in the Green, Amber or Red Zones?

Well-Being

Finally we come to Well-Being.

Really this can make more sense if we turn the phrase around the other way.

Being Well.

This part of our lives is an Overview of how all the parts of our lives are working together.

It is the Reality of our Lives:

> How well we are actually Living, the Quality of our Lives, the Happiness, the Contentment, our Dreams, our Achievements.
>
> It's the Accounting House of Who, How and What we are.

Being Well is about how much Positivity and how much Negativity is in our lives and how this affects us.

Well-Being is often talked about as; A State of Mind.

What State is your mind in?

If you were to think about your Well-Being (or Being Well) and then you were to apply The Dieters Scale© to the different areas of your Well-Being:

> Which parts of your Well-Being would be in the Green, Amber or Red Zones?

So what do I want you to take away from this chapter?

None of us are completed works.

We are all able to make something else of ourselves.

What we need to Be Successful In Our Lives is:

Purpose.
Direction.
A Path to Follow.
Realistic Timescales.
The Correct Application Of Actions.
An Open Mind.

Any persistent weight problem; anywhere on the Spectrum of Weight Problems can be Resolved, Improved or Managed in a better way.

If you can't really do it on your own; get appropriate help.

Chapter 32

Diet, Weight Loss And Exercise Classes

In reality there are lots of Diet and Weight Loss clubs and lots of Exercise classes. So finding one will not be that difficult for most people.

The thing is, that once you have found one:

> How do you avoid doing the same old things once again; and avoid ending up back in the same old place once again?

I guess that the best thing to do is to start looking at this with the question:

> Why do you end up there in the first place?

We can't get away from the simple fact that diet, weight loss and exercise classes exist and that they are big business.

These businesses market themselves to people with weight problems, as being providers of successful weight loss and weight control solutions.

They all hold themselves up as being "The Experts" on the processes of Losing Weight, Maintaining Weight Loss, Getting and Keeping Fit and Living a better quality of life.

And at a surface level this looks to be a fantastic thing; and it's what you really want as well. So it must be a perfect fit!

Well maybe not such a perfect fit as we first think it is. So let's have a better look at this thing and I will give you my view.

They did it and so can you!

In reality; the Holy Grail for Diet, Weight Loss and Exercise providers, is to have someone go through their programmes and to lose lots and lots of weight.

This person is then held up as an example of what can be achieved.

In addition they will often heavily market that persons success at weight loss as a validation for their system.

Those with weight problems will be familiar with this type of marketing.

That simple marketing method of:

They did it; so can you with brand (X) Diet!

And we see a happy, confident, smiling person in all the adverts.

But what happens when we get behind the marketing image and into the everyday reality?

It might be useful if we look at these classes and meetings in another way.

Go through My Gateway and follow My Path!

Let's consider all these different classes and meetings to be Gateways.

Each business, brand and approach is actually a Gateways to a different method of losing weight, getting fitter and feeling better about yourself.

Now as well as being Gateways they are also something else!

Because once you go through a Gateway, you then need a Path to follow, to get you where you want to go to.

So the reality is that the system that you buy into and use on a weekly basis; provides the Path that you will be following and using to achieve and maintain those results you expect.

So the Path that is being provided to you; needs to be able to take you where you want to go to.

> If there is a difference between their marketing hype and their ability to actually deliver what they hype to a mass audience; then this is the reality gap that many of their users will fall into.
>
> The larger the organisation and the more people it needs to attract; the bigger the reality gap is likely to be.

You see many people have been Conditioned to think that diet and weight loss classes, and dieting and weight control products; are the safe and sure route to weight loss and weight control success.

They have also been led to believe that once they achieve weight loss success, that other things will then sort themselves out. And as a result; they will then be able to live better, happier lives as more successful people.

> And all you have to do to achieve the success that you want; is to find the right diet or weight control product.

And billions have been spent on marketing to achieve this "Conditioning of Thinking" for people with problems with their weight over the last few decades.

In order to get a proper understanding of the effectiveness of these providers, I think that you have to look at the thing in a different way.

My way of viewing this would be:

> How many of those who start these Diet, Weight Loss and Exercise classes actually achieve and maintain the results that they wanted to achieve when they began these classes?

And the reality is that we will never know the answer to this question, because no-one will ever provide this information.

It's not in the providers interest to do so!

This is because it is easier to attract people to a big marketing promise; than it is to deliver on that big marketing promise.

For example:

You may attract 10,000,000 people by making big marketing promises. However; it is when it comes time to delivering on those big marketing promises to those 10,000,000 people that the game actually changes. How do they make it a reality?

Now as the scale of overweight people has continued to increase and it has become more difficult to deliver on marketing promises; we have the legends that have been added to the marketing material:

- Can work as part of a calorie controlled diet.
- Lifestyle changes may be required to achieve and maintain longer term results.

So when the diet doesn't work, it wasn't really the fault of the diet. The person didn't do enough to make it work. And sometimes this will be correct and other times it will not be.

Either way this leaves the door open for you to return to the diet, weight control and exercise industry for another attempt at achieving the dream.

Some people will say that; some help is better than no help!

And the reality is that this is not always the case.

The reality is that when people go to these classes and meetings, they have a very mixed variety of "Other Reasons" for doing so.

Many of them will have a short term goal and they will not be thinking long term.

In fact; if you try to tell most people what the real chances of success are with what they are doing and how they are doing it; they will not want to know.

> You have to remember that we are dealing with a problem that has recidivist behaviour, is complicated to deal with, where people often seek quick and easy solutions to complicated and difficult problems.

Now I know that many people will object to my saying this and want to hold up examples of those who have been successful with each and every type of programme.

However; a small number of long term successes is not proof that the classes and meetings work; other than for a small number of people.

And the reality is that if you put enough people through a process; then your chances of finding a success that you can promote increases.

When you are processing millions of people each year, as many of these organisations are, you are bound to have a few successes.

However; replicating that success with a broad base of people is the problem.

> What we want to avoid is creating situations which leads to behaviour such as Yo-Yo Dieting and further dieting disappointments.

The Diet, Weight Control and Exercise Industry are not interested in focusing on the failures of their business; only on the successes.

And in a sense that is the right business thing to do.

However; all businesses should want to improve their products and services. And Diet and Weight loss providers should not be any different.

And this is perhaps where we can see the separation between what the person with a weight problem wants; and what the businesses wants and can actually deliver.

> The businesses aren't selling successful weight loss; they are selling a Possible Way for you to achieve weight loss.
>
> And those who also sell products are selling you more Comfortable ways of doing so while using their products.

In effect many of these businesses rely upon people wanting to lose weight; but their business can't rely upon you losing weight and keeping it off.

> The simple reality is that so much of what makes a difference to the Success or the Failure of someone's life; is outside of the ability of the diet, weight control or exercise plan to influence.

So a question that I would ask is:

What is the actual business of these different Gateways?

What we really need to understand is:

- What is really within the ability of the provider?
- What can they actually deliver to me or help me to really achieve?
- How long will it really take?
- Will they be with me as I go on and undertake this journey to improve my life?

Going down your dream Path.

So you have chosen your diet and weight loss provider and you have signed up and entered through their Gateway.

You are going to attend your first meeting or class and your expectations are high.

Now let's see where you want that Path that you have chosen, to lead you to.

Does it include:

- Weight loss.
- Weight control.
- Want to feel better.
- Want to look better.
- More control over your life.
- Deal with the other issues.
- Looking to improve your life.
- Being more successful in life.

The reality is, that on a monthly basis, there are millions of people using diet and weight loss programmes and exercise classes.

And when you get to the foundation stone for all the different reasons why people are doing so; you find that all of these people have a simple goal in mind:

> They are looking to Improve their lives and be happier than they are. And they are hoping that this will help them do that.

This can appear to be a simple and easy thing

But what we do know is that it is easier to deal with people with lower scale (Green Zone) weight problems, than it is to deal with people with higher scale (Amber and Red Zone) weight problems.

The higher the scale the more difficult, and the less likely that they will achieve success through these classes and meetings.

So once again let's use The Dieters Scale© to help us understand this and see if we can use this to improve success rates.

The questions for this book are:

- Can Diet, Weight Loss and Exercise classes really help you?
- What level and type of problem can they really help with you with?
- Are you being realistic with what you "Really" want to achieve from this process?

My answer to these simple question is going to be one based on my own experiences. It is not going to be based on the different claims made by the many different providers.

Can Diet, Weight Loss and Exercise classes really help you?

If I was working with someone who was on a Life Improvement Programme focused on a Weight Problem; would I have a problem with them using one of these classes?

I have been in the position of having to deal with this and this was and is my view.

I would have concerns over the Expectations that my client currently has and previously had of the dieting industry.

I would be concerned that they would be lured back to promises of easy weight loss when things became difficult in the work that we were doing.

I would want to know what their reasoning was behind wanting to do so at the same time as working with me?

If they were adamant that they did want to do this, then I may agree but with caveats (Terms). I may also say that they need to chose one way or the other.

The reason for this is that although my Life Improvement Programmes and the Diet, Weight Control and Exercise Industry may seem to be in agreement on a number of things:

> The reality is that we are Philosophically different.

We also operate differently, have different tools which we use, understand the problems differently and believe in different types of solutions.

I have expressed my concern over the Timing of the many aspects of dealing with a weight problem.

And about how unforeseen pressures can be put upon the person by themselves. As a result of them thinking that they are doing the right thing, in the right way, at the right time, for the right reasons.

Diet and Exercise classes are one of those things where the timing needs to be right, and the exercise programme also needs to be right.

> You have to remember that we are dealing with a problem that has recidivist behaviour, is complicated to deal with, where people often seek quick and easy solutions to complicated and difficult problems; and failure rates are high.

So if these classes are approached with the right reasons and an appropriate plan; then they could be effective in the right circumstances.

What level and type of problem can they really help with you with?

The answer to this question is difficult because we are going to be working with generalities.

To make this easier we will use The Dieters Scale

to help us understand it better.

We have used The Dieters Scale© to help you begin to see that:

Not all Weight Problems are equal.

And we used The Dieters Scale to grade the level of the different aspects of the weight problem.

So your own weight problem is going to be in either the Green Zone, the Amber Zone or the Red Zone.

In addition to the weight problem there are going to be other aspects of your life which influence and are affected by the weight problem. We can also grade these.

So other things like relationships, for example, may overall be graded Green, Amber or Red. And individual relationships may also be graded Green, Amber or Red.

And through this process we begin to build a Map of the different aspects of your life that form part of your persistent weight problem in one way or another.

> Now what we want to consider is: How much of that Map can be helped by the classes that you are considering attending?

I have done a simple Life Map and it is shown on the next page.

Each circle in the Map represents an aspect of your life and the Zone State that it would currently be in.

In this Map you can see that we have all the Zones represented. The Zones include things like relationships, weight, self-esteem, confidence, etc.

Now if the class you are going to attend is only going to deal with one or two of the Zones that are Green; then how will the other Zones be dealt with?

Do the people have the skills and understanding to actually deal with this type of problem mix?

Your Life Map!

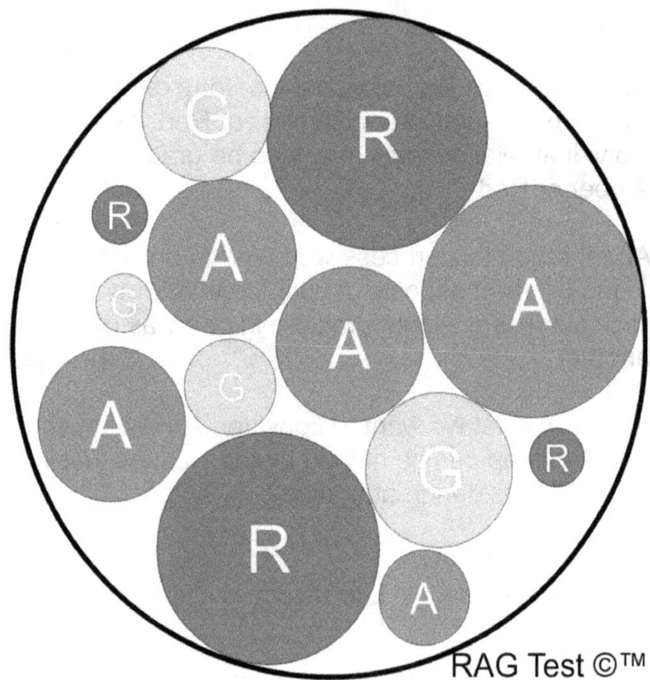

This Map is a simple illustration of the different aspects of a weight problem and the associated issues. Created using The Dieters Scale. The Dieters Scale is part of The Human Dynamics Matrix.

The final questions was:

Are you being realistic with what you "Really" want to achieve from this process?

In the previous question we looked at a simple Life Map. What would your Life Map be like?

Would it be more complicated, have larger Amber Zones or be more or less all one colour?

Consider what your Life Map might be like and then answer the question.

> Are you being realistic with what you "Really" want to achieve from this process?

Over the years I have had to watch many different people make mistakes and get things wrong.

Sometimes it was little things and other times it was big things.

When you deal with problems like alcohol and drug addiction, and long term weight problems that severely impact someone's life and other life problems: You often see that things could have been different if someone had only done (X) at a certain point in time.

You can see that what they needed to do (X) was Often within their capability; but they don't do it. My final point is one that should be within your capability to appreciate and understand:

> If the solution that you are considering does not match the needs of the problem; then it is very unlikely to work!
>
> If that is the case; why are you considering it?

So what do I want you to take away from this chapter?

> All problems have a structure that can be understood.
>
> All solutions have a structure that can be understood.
>
> The better the fit between the two; the more successful the outcome can be.

I hope that you have found this book to be interesting and that it has made you think about things in a different and productive way.

If it has; please recommend it to someone else!

David John Sheridan aka Guru David

About Guru David

Life would be great if it was perfect. Unfortunately life often falls short of perfection and often lacks clarity.

How do we make a better life in an imperfect world with lots of competing pressures?

Nature provides us with a lot of gifts that we can use to experience Life and to help us to be successful in whatever environment that we find ourselves in.

Unfortunately these gifts do not come with instructions and we need to learn through experience how to understand, interpret and manage these wonderful gifts.

Nature does not provide us with instruction manuals but it does provide us with special people who are able to help us with living our lives and making our living experiences the best that they can be.

Guru David is one of these special people.

Why would someone want to use a Guru?

Guru's tend to live a different life to normal people. They have different life experiences and they think and behave differently.

Guru's will often have encountered and overcome many types of hardships and difficulties. These will often be physical and cerebral and can occur over long periods of time, often decades.

Guru's will understand Humanity and Human Nature better and they often have insights and understanding of things that others do not.

Guru's make good guides, advisors and mentors when difficult, complex and challenging issues have to be addressed. They provide confidentiality and support as appropriate and help to achieve clarity of thoughts and actions.

A good Guru deals with reality and understands societies structures and pressures.

Meet an extra ordinary person

Guru David creates custom approaches for challenges that involve Feelings, Emotions, Psychology, Behaviours, Experiences, Knowledge and acquired Wisdom.

Guru David accepts selected personal and business clients that he feels that he can work with.

Guru David's approach includes using The Way of Vartis and his authoritative work with The Human Algorithm® Project.

A graduate of The College of The Richmond Fellowship; an experienced counsellor and therapist with specialist training, knowledge and experience of Alcohol and Drug Addiction with a high level of knowledge and experience working with dependency issues, problem architecture, problem dynamics and related Human Algorithm's®.

Guru David is an authority on working with Obesity and Weight Control issues and provides a customised approach that includes work from his books covering this subject.

Due to his work with problem architecture, problem dynamics and Human Algorithm's, Guru David is well placed to understand many different problem types and provide help to develop effective solution focused approaches.

Guru David's other books include understanding Motivation; working with Self Esteem and The Human Dynamics Matrix.

Guru David's other experiences and knowledge include obtaining black belts in martial arts, experienced in working with finance and debt resolution for members of the public, business consultancy, different levels of training, writing books and articles, being targeted by trolls, being victimised and abused for having a different view and behaviours, being targeted and the victim of financial crimes, experience around the music industry, innovation, design, building and an interest in different types of engineering, construction, physics and nature.

At different times, Guru David's resilience has inspired and amazed others and frustrated those who have tried to destroy him and his work.

Guru David has other knowledge, experiences and wisdom that can be revealed and shared at appropriate times.

Guru David would describe himself as spiritual rather than religious and this is evident in The Way of Vartis.

The Way of Vartis offers a view of the celestial reality of the universe, the truth about the future, the knowledge that people need to change how they live within their personal environments and the honesty of the reality of Life and why we are here.

The Way of Vartis provides an open approach and does not impose dogma. As a result someone can choose to add The Way of Vartis to their life and achieve the benefits without being required to give up any religious practices or beliefs they hold.

Guru David can be hired or consulted for specific or more general work.

Those who are interested in supporting The Way of Vartis or The Human Algorithm® Project can become a follower, supporter or sponsor.

Guru David can work in a variety of countries by arrangement and is comfortable to work through good quality interpreters.

Hello Readers!

You can find more information about the things that I am doing by visiting the following websites:

www.gurudavid.co.uk

www.vartis.co.uk

You can email me; Guru David with any comments or inquiries at: david@gurudavid.co.uk

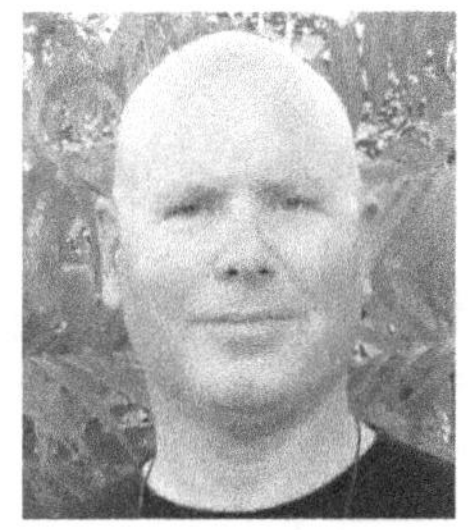

www.ingramcontent.com/pod-product-compliance
Lightning Source LLC
Chambersburg PA
CBHW062158270326
41930CB00009B/1578
9780993235535